A Com
Preventi

SURVIVAL

OF THE

CLEANEST

Jacob I. T. van der Merwe

Spicers
Publishing

Disclaimer:
This book is intended as a guide to preventive hygiene, not as a medical manual, first aid manual or guide to self-treatment; nor is it intended to offer medical advice in any way. Always consult with a doctor or other qualified healthcare professional if you have a medical problem or if you require information on health-related matters. The author and publishers are not responsible for any problems that may develop from the use or misuse of the information provided in this book.

Copyright © 2005 by Jacob I. T. van der Merwe

All rights reserved. No part of this book may be reproduced or transmitted in any form or by any means, electronic or mechanical, including photocopying, recording, or by any information storage and retrieval system, without prior permission in writing from the publisher.

Canadian Cataloguing in Publication Data

Van der Merwe, Jacob I. T., 1962-
    Survival of the Cleanest : A Common Sense Guide to
    Preventing Infectious Disease.

ISBN 0-9739201-0-6

    1. Hygiene.   2. Self-care, Health.   I. Title.
RA643.V36 2005   613   C2005-907332-2

Spicers Publishing
Victoria, BC
V8P 1M7 Canada

spicerspublishing.com

Printed in Canada

FOR CHRISTINE

CONTENTS

Introduction	7
Basic Rules	14
Public Washrooms	42
Food Safety	54
Motor Vehicles	81
Public Transportation	83
Workplace Hygiene	88
Public Telephones, ABMs & Shared Computers	92
Shopping	99
Medical Facilities	108
Recreational Facilities	122
Travel	129
Camping & Outdoors	157
Drinking Water	182
Hygiene in the Home	200
Pets & Wild Animals	222
Insects	236
Gardening	252
Litter	261
Germ Etiquette	264
New Technology to the Rescue?	267
Index	278

INTRODUCTION

Forty years ago, the threat of infectious disease appeared to be waning. New vaccines, antibiotic drugs, improved sanitation technology, and other scientific advances had led to the control and prevention of many infectious diseases. Deaths from infection, commonplace at the beginning of the twentieth century, were no longer a frequent occurrence in developed countries. Chemical pesticides like DDT were lowering the incidence of insect-borne diseases such as malaria, and by the early 1960's insect-borne disease was no longer regarded as a major threat to global public health.

The world was enjoying a vacation from infectious disease. But the vacation was about to end.

Today, new infectious diseases are emerging and existing diseases thought to be under control are re-emerging. There is a resurgence of infectious diseases throughout the world, including outbreaks of typhoid, cholera, malaria and yellow fever. The number of people infected with the human immunodeficiency virus (HIV) that causes AIDS has reached 40 million and continues to increase in many countries. More than 20 million people have died of AIDS since 1981. The Ebola virus, which causes a fatal haemorrhagic fever, has appeared

INTRODUCTION

again in Africa. Recurring outbreaks of avian influenza (bird flu) in Asia continue to take a deadly toll and threaten to cause a worldwide epidemic on a scale never seen before in history.

It is impossible to turn on the television, browse a news web site or open a newspaper without encountering reports about bird flu, mad cow disease, West Nile virus, Norwalk virus, outbreaks of *E. coli*, *Salmonella* or some newly discovered pathogen. The 2003 outbreak of Severe Acute Respiratory Syndrome (SARS) killed 774 people worldwide in less than eight months. Deadly outbreaks of Marburg haemorrhagic fever and bubonic plague are becoming increasingly difficult to contain and experts fear that they could spread globally. Insect-borne diseases are also re-emerging.

New diseases have appeared within North America, including SARS, Lyme disease, Legionnaire's disease and West Nile disease. Other new or re-emerging threats in North America include drug-resistant tuberculosis; antibiotic-resistant bacteria that cause pneumonia, meningitis and flesh-eating disease; as well as diarrheal diseases caused by parasites and by several strains of *E. coli* bacteria.

Several factors contribute to the increase in incidence of infectious diseases:

- population shifts and population growth;
- changes in human behaviour;
- urbanization;
- poverty;

INTRODUCTION

- overcrowding;
- political instability;
- changes in ecology and climate;
- evolution and mutation of microbes;
- inadequate public health infrastructures;
- modern travel and global trade.

For example, the speed of modern travel means outbreaks of disease in remote areas can quickly spread to crowded urban areas. In the 1300s, it took three years for bubonic plague to get from southern Italy to Britain. Today, it would take only a few hours. Thanks to world travel, exotic infections are becoming commonplace. We cannot build up resistance fast enough against this changing array of pathogens.

Behavioural factors such as eating habits, personal hygiene, unprotected sex and intravenous drug use can contribute to the spread of disease. Human encroachment on tropical forests has brought people into close contact with insects that carry malaria, yellow fever and other insect-borne diseases. Changes in temperature and rainfall affect the number of germ-carrying rodents in some areas.

Political instability leads to wars that destroy health and food distribution infrastructures. Refugees end up in camps where crowded and unsanitary conditions create the perfect environment for infectious diseases to spread. Economic instability leads to mass migration, across and within international borders, often into crowded urban areas. Basic public health services, such

INTRODUCTION

as nutrition and vaccination programs cannot keep up with exploding city populations. Overcrowding places a burden on water supplies, sewage systems and garbage removal, further increasing the likelihood of disease outbreaks.

Viruses and bacteria mutate at an ever-increasing rate, making it impossible for our immune systems to keep up. Scientists are worried about more diseases crossing the species barrier and becoming contagious among humans. Many of these germs could remain in strains against which people have no natural resistance. Antibiotic-resistant bacteria are commonplace.

Not only are we faced with more harmful microbes, but the resulting infections are also becoming increasingly deadly and devastating. Outbreaks of these terrible diseases cause widespread fear and panic. People feel helpless; they expect their governments to protect them and their families from harm. They expect immediate and effective safety measures.

The truth is, it is impossible for any government to protect all of its citizens against every infectious disease all the time. Even if they can prevent, control or eradicate major outbreaks of deadly infectious diseases like SARS and bird flu, we're still left to protect ourselves against the myriad of other infections that, even though they don't always cause large-scale epidemics, can be equally deadly to the infected individual.

Infectious diseases are the leading cause of death worldwide. Diseases like meningitis, dysentery, viral pneumonia, typhoid, hepatitis, infectious diarrhea, strep throat, seasonal flu, malaria and cholera continue to

INTRODUCTION

infect millions of people around the globe. Everybody is at risk, irrespective of whether you live in a developing country, or in North America or Europe.

All infectious diseases have three things in common:

- they are caused by germs;
- infection is a mechanical process that requires germs to enter the body; and
- the mechanics of infection can be disrupted.

Infection takes place when bacteria, viruses, fungi or parasites enter the body and begin to multiply. **Disease** occurs when cells in the body are damaged because of the infection, and symptoms of an illness appear.

We can take a number of steps to prevent infection from occurring in the first place:

- **Preventive medication:** Some medicines can protect us from infectious germs. For example, taking antiparasitic medication might protect us from contracting malaria if we travel to a region where the risk of infection is high. After exposure to certain bacteria, such as those that cause bacterial meningitis, taking antibiotics may lower our risk of infection. Over-the-counter antibiotic creams or ointments can be used for minor cuts and scrapes. However, long-term, indiscriminate use of antibiotics is not recommended. It won't prevent bacterial infections and may result in more resistant strains of bacteria when infections do occur. All medications have side effects, and some can be severe. Preventive medicines

INTRODUCTION

should only be taken when there is a clear danger of exposure to serious disease and, as a last resort, when other measures fail to provide full protection.

- **Vaccination:** Vaccination can prevent a number of diseases. The list of vaccine-preventable diseases continues to grow. Many vaccines are administered in childhood, but adults still need to be routinely vaccinated to prevent some illnesses, such as tetanus and influenza. While generally regarded as safe, vaccination is not without risk. Like other medications, vaccines can cause unwanted side effects in some people. Vaccination should not be our first or only line of defence against infection.
- **Preventive hygiene:** Our best defence is to avoid the germs that cause infection. Improved cleanliness is the easiest, least expensive and most effective way to protect ourselves from most infections. Unlike medicines and vaccines, it has no side effects. Incredibly, many people remain ignorant of the dangers and do not take the most basic precautions to prevent the spread of infectious diseases. Several studies show that as many as one in five people do not even wash their hands after using the bathroom, one of the easiest and most effective ways to avoid infection and stop germs from spreading. Diligence, knowledge, and a common sense approach to preventive hygiene are our main weapons in the fight against the spread of everything from the common cold to more serious diseases such as hepatitis and Severe Acute Respiratory Syndrome (SARS).

INTRODUCTION

About the Book

Survival of the Cleanest is a comprehensive and practical guide to preventive hygiene. The first chapter covers the basic, universally applicable rules for preventing infectious disease. The remaining chapters deal with specific topics, including public washrooms, food safety, public transportation, workplace hygiene, shopping, medical facilities, travel, germ etiquette, the solutions offered by new technology, and more.

The book is designed to be used as a quick reference guide: Feel free to go directly to the chapters that interest you most, or use the comprehensive index provided at the back of the book.

BASIC RULES

To avoid infection, we first need to understand how germs spread. Germs can be transported into the body by one of several mechanisms.

Many infections are caused by indirect contact when our hands transfer germs from contaminated objects, such as doorhandles, raw meat, cutting boards and cleaning cloths, to susceptible parts of the body. Our hands touch many surfaces in the course of a day. They are prime vehicles for transferring germs to our noses, mouths and eyes, or to objects and surfaces where they can be passed on to other people. With very few exceptions, most germs can be transmitted in this way.

We can also become infected when we inhale small particles, dust and water droplets that are contaminated with germs. Pathogens get into the respiratory tract via the nose and mouth. Diseases like influenza (flu), measles, and tuberculosis are transmitted this way.

Several serious infectious diseases, including hepatitis A, cholera, polio, salmonellosis and dysentery propagate through the ingestion of contaminated food and water.

Infection can also occur when germs enter the body through cuts, scratches, injections, animal and insect bites, burns or other wounds to the skin and mucous membranes. Malaria, septicemia, tetanus, Lyme disease, hepatitis B, and methicillin-resistant *Staphylococcus aureus* (MRSA) are transmitted this way.

And finally, infections such as gonorrhoea, herpes simplex type two and HIV/AIDS are passed on through sexual contact between partners.

There are **13 Basic Rules** of preventive hygiene. Following these rules will dramatically reduce your risk of infection.

Know the Enemy

Infectious diseases are caused by various types of microscopic germs, also referred to as pathogens. Germs are divided into four main groups: bacteria, viruses, fungi and parasites.

- **Bacteria** are microscopic one-celled organisms, found in the human body, in animals and everywhere in the environment. Many bacteria can survive in adverse conditions. Some can withstand extreme heat or cold; others can survive radiation levels that would be lethal to humans and animals. They multiply by subdivision and most are self-sufficient; they do not need a host to survive. Some bacteria, known as infectious bacteria, cause disease. Bacteria are responsible for a wide range of infectious diseases, including food poisoning, diarrhea, septicemia, pneumonia, staph infection, strep throat, skin infections, eye infections, urinary tract infections, botulism and anthrax. When infectious bacteria enter the body they multiply and release toxins into the body. The toxins damage the cells they have invaded, causing illness or an infection. Bacteria can spread via contaminated surfaces such as doorhandles and toilet seats, contaminated food or drinks, blood and other body fluids, sexual contact and lack of hygiene. Bacteria are classified by their shapes. Spherical bacteria are called *cocci*, rod-shaped bacteria are called *bacilli*, and spiral-shaped or helical bacteria are called *spirochetes*.

- **Viruses** are the smallest members of the germ family. They can only be seen with an electron microscope. A virus has one main objective, and that is to reproduce. Viruses are not self-sufficient; they need a suitable host to reproduce. A virus is basically a container for DNA or RNA genetic material. DNA or RNA is the genetic code containing the information needed to replicate the virus. When a virus invades the body, it enters and takes over a number of cells. It instructs the host cells to manufacture the elements it needs to reproduce. The host cells are usually destroyed in the process. Examples of viral diseases include the common cold, flu, hepatitis, smallpox, West Nile virus, bird flu, encephalitis, SARS, rabies, Norwalk virus, hantavirus, polio and HIV/AIDS.

Viruses are transmitted in a number of ways. They can be swallowed with contaminated food or drinks, inhaled, picked up from contaminated surfaces, some are sexually transmitted, and others are transmitted by the bites of insects and parasites. Blood and other body fluids are also effective carriers for viruses.

BASIC RULES

- Most **Fungi** are single-celled organisms that are somewhat larger than bacteria. Yeast and mold are examples of single-celled fungi. Fungi are found everywhere. They live in the air, water, soil and on plants. They can live in our bodies, mostly without making us sick. Some fungi even have beneficial uses. The antibiotic penicillin is derived from fungi. Fungi are also essential in making certain foods, such as bread, cheese, yogurt, beer and wine.
However, some fungi are not benign and can cause infection and illness. Some of the more common types of fungal infections are tinea (ringworm), a fungal infection of the hair, skin, or nails; athlete's foot, a fungal infection between the toes or on the feet; and jock itch, a fungal infection of the groin area. Another example is candida, a yeast that causes thrush, an infection of the mouth and throat; diaper rash; and yeast infection in and around the vagina. Many fungal infections are contagious, which means they easily spread from person to person. Close contact or sharing clothes, a comb or a hairbrush with someone who has a fungal infection can spread the fungus from one person to another. Because fungi need a warm and humid place to grow, public showers, pools, and locker rooms provide the perfect environment for fungi to spread.
- **Parasites** are organisms that can live inside the human body, in animals and birds, and in insects. Parasites that can infect people are divided into two groups: *Protozoa* and *Helminths*.

Protozoa are single-celled organisms that can live inside the body as parasites. Some protozoa live in the intestinal tract and are quite harmless. Others cause serious diseases such as cryptosporidiosis, or crypto, a diarrheal disease caused by *Cryptosporidium* parasites; giardiasis, a diarrheal illness caused by *Giardia* parasites; and malaria. They can spend part of their life cycle outside human or animal hosts, living in food, soil, water or insects. Protozoa can be ingested with food or drinking water, spread through sexual contact or propagate via vectors, meaning they rely on other organisms to spread from person to person. Malaria is an example of a disease caused by a vector-borne parasite, mosquitoes being the vector for the malaria parasite.

The word *helminth* means worm. The most common helminths are tapeworms and roundworms. When helminths or their eggs get inside the body, they settle in the intestinal tract, lungs, liver, skin or brain, living off the nutrients in the body. Roundworms can range in length from 15 to 35 centimetres; some tapeworms can grow to seven metres or longer. A tapeworm has hundreds of segments, each of which can break off and develop into a new tapeworm.

Recognize the Danger Zones

Danger zones are areas and objects where there are both high concentrations of dangerous germs and the possibility that they will be passed on to others. The

BASIC RULES

most common danger zones are listed below. This is by no means meant to be a complete list; harmful germs are everywhere.

- public washrooms
- food service outlets
- litter
- pets and wild animals
- money
- public phones
- computer keyboards
- toilet seats
- telephones
- workout equipment
- tanning beds
- swimming pools
- hot tubs
- rental shoes
- grocery cart handles
- theaters
- waiting rooms
- elevators
- remote controls
- game controllers
- banking machines
- gas pumps
- doorhandles
- public showers
- public sinks
- bowling balls
- slot machines
- water fountains
- cruise ships
- aircraft
- subways
- buses
- taxi cabs
- trains
- hotels
- motels
- casinos
- offices
- health clubs
- nursing homes
- day care centres
- dentists' offices
- doctors' offices
- clinics
- hospitals
- schools
- dormitories
- amusement parks

SURVIVAL OF THE CLEANEST

- restaurants
- bars
- night clubs
- lobbies
- microphones
- rental cars
- government offices
- grocery stores
- pharmacies
- any public area

Keep Your Hands Clean

This is the most effective and important precaution in the fight against infectious disease. It may seem like stating the obvious, but you will be surprised (and shocked) by how many people fail to keep their hands sufficiently clean to prevent contracting and spreading infectious germs. By frequently washing our hands, we remove the germs we picked up from other people, from contaminated surfaces, from animals, and other sources. The US Centers for Disease Control and Prevention (CDC) considers hand washing to be the single most important means of preventing the spread of infection.

If we do not keep our hands clean, we pick up germs from other sources and then infect ourselves when we:

- eat, prepare or handle food;
- touch our eyes, noses, mouths or genitals;
- touch any areas of broken skin, such as cuts, sores, burns or acne.

We can also spread germs directly to others or onto surfaces that other people touch. And before we know it, everybody around us is getting sick. According to the

BASIC RULES

CDC, each year 10 to 20 percent of US residents contract the flu, more than 100,000 are hospitalized, and an average of 36,000 actually die from the disease. An estimated 1,500 people die from the flu each year in Canada.

Hand washing is an effective and inexpensive weapon against the spread of flu viruses. In addition to colds and the flu, other serious diseases, like hepatitis A, meningitis, SARS, Norwalk virus, infectious diarrhea and other gastrointestinal and respiratory illnesses can easily be prevented if people make a habit of keeping their hands clean.

We keep our hands clean by doing two things:

- by avoiding contamination in the first place; and
- by washing them frequently and thoroughly.

You may find yourself thinking: 'What's the big deal? Everybody over the age of two does this as a matter of habit.' Sadly, this is not true. There are numerous studies that show that people are a lot less diligent about washing their hands than we would like to believe. It is estimated that one out of every five people do not wash their hands after using the washroom. And even those who wash their hands regularly quite often don't do a very good job.

A survey done in 2003 by the American Society for Microbiology (ASM) found that more than one in five people neglect to wash their hands after using airport restrooms. The ASM put observers in airport washrooms at six major airports in North America. A total of 7,539 men and women were observed either washing or not washing their hands in New York City, San Francisco, Chicago, Dallas, Miami and Toronto. Incredibly, 22 percent of the people observed didn't wash their hands before leaving the washrooms.

Still not convinced? Try this experiment. Go to the washroom at the airport, at work or any public washroom with reasonably high traffic. Hang around unobtrusively for ten minutes. Find a spot where you can observe the washbasins. Take note of the following:

- people who use the washroom and leave without washing their hands at all;
- those who just rinse their hands without going near the soap;
- those who use soap, but spend only two or three seconds on the entire process; and
- observe those people who wash their hands really thoroughly, and see how they go about drying their hands.

Let us hope that, should you conduct this experiment at your favourite restaurant, you do not see the chef, or your waiter, use the washroom without washing his or her hands!

You may argue that if people choose not to wash their hands properly it is their business, and they harm only themselves. Not true. People who don't wash their hands properly not only run the risk of infecting themselves; they also deposit their germs on any surface they touch, ready to infect the next unsuspecting individual. That

BASIC RULES

means we have to be even more vigilant about keeping our own hands clean and germ-free.

Now that we realize that everybody isn't necessarily diligent about washing their hands, the first thing we need to do is to avoid touching contaminated objects as far as possible. It is, of course, quite impossible to go through life without touching anything. The solution is to avoid *direct* contact with objects and surfaces that are likely to be contaminated.

Public washroom doorhandles are perfect examples. They are guaranteed to be germ-infested. You never, ever want to touch a doorknob in a public toilet with your bare hands. Always use a paper towel or any available barrier to protect your hands when opening a washroom door.

Also avoid directly touching any surfaces in high-traffic areas, such as escalator rails, elevator buttons, doorhandles and others. Recent outbreaks of the Norwalk virus on cruise ships were traced back to infected individuals who touched doorhandles without washing their hands thoroughly. Contrary to popular belief, the number of cold and flu infections caused by airborne viruses are actually relatively few. Most people contract colds and flu through contact with contaminated surfaces and then touching their mouths, eyes, noses or food. The SARS virus is another recent example of a pathogen that spreads easily via contaminated surfaces and objects.

It goes without saying that shaking hands with other people is a risky activity. I am not suggesting that we stop greeting other people with a handshake. This is another situation that calls for a common sense approach. If shaking hands is required or unavoidable, wash your hands as soon as is practical without offending the other party. Be careful not to touch your nose, mouth, eyes, any areas of broken skin or genitals.

The reality is that we use our hands to handle and touch objects and surfaces, we greet other people with a handshake, and we have to go to the bathroom. Correctly washing our hands therefore becomes the single most important step we can take to protect ourselves from infectious disease.

Three basic principles apply to washing your hands:

- wash your hands frequently;
- wash them correctly and thoroughly; and
- do not recontaminate your hands after washing.

Wash Frequently

Washing our hands frequently means washing as often as we can. For most people this probably means washing their hands more often than they do now. Germs aren't visible to the naked eye; nor can we smell or feel them, so germs may be present on hands that appear to be perfectly clean.

Wash your hands whenever they may have been exposed to germs. At a minimum, always wash your hands:

- before eating;
- before, during and after preparing or handling food;

BASIC RULES

- after eating;
- after using the bathroom;
- before using the toilet;
- after changing a diaper;
- after contact with blood or other body fluids like vomit, nasal secretions or saliva;
- before administering medicines;
- before and after having sex;
- before and after changing a tampon;
- before putting in contact lenses;
- before and after treating a wound;
- after changing a cat's litter box;
- after touching a rubbish bin or drain;
- after touching a cleaning cloth;
- after touching a contaminated surface;
- after shaking hands;
- after shopping;
- after handling pets, other animals or animal waste;
- before and after brushing teeth;
- before applying or touching up make-up;
- after gardening;
- after opening mail;
- after handling money;
- after using public transportation;
- when your hands are dirty;
- after blowing your nose;
- after coughing or sneezing;

- more frequently when you are sick;
- more frequently when someone at home is sick;
- after handling raw meat, fish or poultry;
- after picking up an object from the floor;
- after taking out the garbage;
- after touching any part of your body;
- after clearing tables and handling dirty dishes, pots, pans and cooking utensils;
- after using household cleaners; and
- as often in between as you can.

Wash Correctly and Thoroughly

Washing our hands correctly and thoroughly is as important, if not more so, than washing them frequently. Unfortunately, many people do not follow the correct steps when washing their hands. Again, just observe what other people do next time you are in a public washroom. I don't know why some people even bother; sometimes the effort is not worth the water wasted.

It is important to understand that washing your hands is a mechanical process. While the hot water and the chemical action of the soap will kill some of the germs, the primary effect of washing your hands is the mechanical removal of dirt and germs from the skin's surface. To ensure that all contaminants are removed from your hands, follow the steps below:

- **Use clean, hot running water** – Let the water run as hot as you can stand without scalding the skin. Using hot water serves three *purposes: it does a better job dissolving dirt and grime than cold water; some germs are killed by the sudden change in temperature; and many soaps foam, activate and clean better with hot water.*

- **Rinse hands thoroughly** – Rinse your hands from about two inches above the wrists to the fingertips, turning them in the hot water stream to remove any loose dirt and to prepare the skin's surface for the soap. Remove dirt from underneath the fingernails.

- **Apply liquid or clean bar soap** – If you are using liquid soap, squirt a generous amount of soap into the palm of one hand. I do not recommend using bar soap in any public washroom facility, or even at home where a bathroom is shared by several family members. If bar soap is the only option available to you, rinse the bar in hot running water for at least 30 seconds before using it. Rub the bar between your hands until a visible lather forms. Rinse the bar when you're done and place it on a rack or porous surface and allow it to drain.

- **Scrub** – Rub your hands vigorously together and scrub all surfaces, starting about two inches above the wrists down to the fingertips. Be sure to remove any dirt from underneath the fingernails and between the fingers. Continue for at least 30 seconds. Slowly count to 30, recite the alphabet, whistle a short tune, do whatever works for you, as long us you scrub energetically for at least 30 seconds. Remember, it is the scrubbing action, combined with the soap and hot water, that dislodges and removes germs.

- **Rinse with clean, hot running water** – Rinse for at least 15 seconds. Inspect your hands to ensure that no traces of soap or dirt are left on the skin.
- **Repeat** – You won't find this step in any of the conventional recommendations for personal hygiene. It is unfortunate, because this simple, common sense measure provides significant additional protection against contracting infectious disease. There are those who would argue that this is overkill. First of all, there is nothing wrong with overkill when your health or your family's safety is at stake. That said, if we examine the logic, we will see that this is not a superfluous measure, but a necessary step in ridding our hands of harmful micro-organisms and other contaminants. This step adds redundancy to the process: any germs we miss the first time around, we get the next. It's as simple as that and worth the extra effort.
- **Final rinse** – Rinse for at least 15 seconds. Inspect your hands to ensure that no traces of soap or dirt are left on the skin.
- **Dry your hands** – The importance of proper drying methods is often overlooked. It is during this step that people frequently recontaminate their hands by not following basic and common sense rules. The first rule is to never use a linen towel in a public washroom. This holds true for traditional cloth towels and the rolls of linen towel found in wall-mounted dispensers. Always assume that reusable towels are not clean or properly disinfected. It is acceptable to use

linen towels at home, as long as each family member uses his or her own hand and body towels. It goes without saying that towels should be changed and washed regularly, preferably daily. In public washrooms, use only warm air dryers or paper towels from a dispenser. Paper towel dispensers that have to be manually operated by means of a lever pose a contamination risk because of people touching the dispensing lever. The way to use them safely is to dispense a paper towel before you wash your hands. After washing your hands, use this paper towel to close the faucet and to dispense more paper towels without directly touching the handle. Thorough hand drying also checks the spread of disease by keeping hands from becoming dry and chapped. Dry and cracked skin provides a surface that is easier for germs to adhere to.

Avoid Recontamination

It makes no sense to carefully wash your hands, only to recontaminate them immediately afterwards by touching unclean surfaces. Sadly, this is the rule, not the exception. How many people avoid directly touching the faucets, doorhandles and paper towel dispensers in public washrooms? Do you? Follow the three golden rules for avoiding recontamination: *As discussed above, use caution when operating paper towel dispensers; always use a paper towel to protect your hands when opening and closing faucets; and use a paper towel as a barrier when touching doorhandles.* I always keep a few heavy-duty facial tissues handy to dry my hands, and to open and close doors and faucets, in case paper towels or air dryers are not available. Wherever doors open away from me I always push them open with my shoe. In an emergency, roll off a few layers of toilet paper to dry your hands and to open the door. This is much safer than using a linen towel or touching the doorhandle with your bare hands.

I also recommend using instant hand sanitizers. Buy sanitizing gels that contain at least 62% ethyl alcohol as the active ingredient. Alcohol is a safe, fast-acting disinfectant that kills most common germs on contact. Sanitizers provide an extra level of protection and peace of mind. I keep a bottle in the car, one on my desk and several of the smaller pocket-sized ones stashed all over the place, including in jacket pockets and in my briefcase. I always use hand sanitizer after having used a public washroom, irrespective of how clean and well-equipped the facility is, or how carefully I've washed and dried my hands. I like the extra insurance! Of course, they are also great to use when you are not able to wash your hands. They are very effective for disinfecting hands and provide a high level of protection.

However, using sanitizers is not a substitute for proper hand washing. While sanitizing gels will kill off many germs, they do not remove dirt from the hands and may not kill some tough viruses such as hepatitis A. If you have to use a sanitizer instead of washing your hands, be sure to wash your hands thoroughly at the earliest opportunity. Antibacterial wipes also work well. Choose those brands that list benzethonium chloride, benzalkonium chloride or alcohol as active ingredients.

They offer the added benefit of mechanically removing surface contaminants in addition to killing germs.

Both sanitizing gels and wipes are fantastic for travel. I actually found that I stopped contracting colds or flu during long-haul flights since I started using the wipes and sanitizers. This proves the connection between clean hands and staying healthy.

The Great Antibacterial Soap Debate

There is a continuing debate about whether or not we should be using antibacterial soaps. Do they offer added protection? Are they safe to use? Do they cause resistant bacteria to develop as a number of controversial studies suggest? Do they work as advertised or are they merely placebos that cause long-term harm to our health and the environment?

Truth be told, as long as you wash your hands correctly and frequently, it probably makes no difference whether you use antibacterial soap or not. Washing your hands is a mechanical process that, if done properly, removes dirt and germs from the skin's surface. Whether or not to use antibacterial soap is a matter of personal preference.

I like the extra protection against bacteria that antibacterial soaps offer, and I do not buy into the theory that the antibacterial ingredients in soap and other cleaners cause resistant bacteria strains. *Triclosan* is the most widely used active ingredient in antibacterial soaps. In the more than 35 years that antibacterial products containing triclosan have been used by consumers and health professionals, triclosan has never been shown to promote antibacterial or antibiotic resistance. In fact, hospitals use antibacterial products every day to stop the spread of bacteria, including drug-resistant bacteria.

Antibacterial soaps contain an active ingredient that keeps the number of germs at a reduced level for an extended period of time, providing improved germ control. Antibacterial products should be used where the level of sanitation is critical and additional precautions are needed to prevent the spread of disease, such as at hospitals, clinics, restaurants, day care centres, schools and other environments where high concentrations of infectious bacteria may be present. They should always be used at home when someone is sick, or when a family member has a compromised immune system.

The active ingredients in antibacterial soap work by penetrating the bacteria's cell walls, thereby neutralizing the bacteria's abilities to function, grow and reproduce. Triclosan and triclocarban are the two ingredients most commonly used in antibacterial soaps. Both have proved to be effective against a wide range of bacteria.

Using antibacterial soap does not mean we can abandon proper hand washing technique. Most of the active ingredients in the antibacterial soap have to be in contact with the bacteria for at least 30 seconds to have the desired effect. Always remember that the primary benefit from washing your hands comes from mechanically removing dirt and germs, no matter what kind of soap you use. Antibacterial soap will not kill some viruses, fungi and parasites.

BASIC RULES

A Word of Caution

Some people are sensitive or allergic to one or more of the active ingredients commonly used in antibacterial soaps. If you develop any kind of skin irritation, rash, excessively dry skin or other adverse reaction, stop using the product immediately! Switch to a different product or regular soap. A rash, excessive dryness or any form of skin irritation compromises the integrity of the skin and its ability to block germs, and leaves you vulnerable to infection. By using a product that irritates the skin you do yourself more harm than good.

To conclude, I strongly believe that it should be made compulsory to use and provide liquid antibacterial soap in public washrooms, schools, restaurants or any place where food is prepared or served to the public. In addition, there should be minimum standards for the type and concentration of the active antibacterial ingredient or, preferably ingredients, for soaps used in these facilities.

A Final Thought on Clean Hands

We not only keep ourselves healthier by keeping our hands clean, but we also avoid spreading germs around that can make others sick. Just imagine how wonderfully clean and healthy the world would be if everyone followed the steps above and kept their hands clean. Imagine being able to touch any surface, go to work, attend school or visit a relative in hospital without the fear of contracting some dreadful disease.

SURVIVAL OF THE CLEANEST

Don't Touch Your Face

Even clean hands should stay away from eyes, noses and mouths to prevent germs from infecting the body. Avoid touching your face and teach children to do the same. This simple precaution can go a long way towards protecting you from colds, the flu, and most eye and skin infections. Don't bite your fingernails or pick your nose; both are guaranteed ways of ingesting germs.

Control Your Environment

The next basic precaution is to keep your immediate environment germ-free. To achieve this you must routinely clean and disinfect surface areas where you live, work and relax. Cleaning and disinfecting are not the same thing. In most cases, cleaning with soap and water is adequate. It removes dirt and most of the germs. However, in other situations disinfecting provides an extra margin of safety.

You should disinfect areas where there are both high concentrations of dangerous germs and a possibility that they will be spread to others. Disinfectants have ingredients that destroy bacteria and other germs. While surfaces may look clean, many infectious germs may be lurking around. Given the right conditions some germs can live on surfaces for hours and even days.

Understanding where the high-risk areas are is an important first step in eliminating harmful germs from your surroundings. Survival of the Cleanest is your comprehensive reference guide to all these hazards.

Avoid Crowds

Whenever possible, avoid places where large groups of people congregate. More people equate to more germs being spread around, thus increasing the odds for infection. This rule applies year-round, but becomes more important during flu season, or whenever an infectious disease is present in your community.

Unless it's an emergency, stay clear of the waiting room at doctors' offices or clinics. Shop during off-peak hours or in smaller, less busy stores. Online shopping is a great way to avoid crowds not only during peak times, but also year-round. Think twice before visiting places where sick kids might be allowed to run free. When crowds can't be avoided, exercise caution and use common sense to avoid infection. Be careful about touching anything, keep your hands clean, don't touch your face and stay clear of people who sneeze and cough.

Never Share Eating or Drinking Utensils

There is nothing romantic or cool about sharing a drink from the same glass with someone else, or using the same fork or spoon. I'd like to believe that most people don't share eating or drinking utensils, at least not with people they are not also willing to kiss. Because that is exactly what it comes down to. If you share a drinking glass or fork with another person, you share his or her saliva and all the germs that thrive in that medium.

The other thing to bear in mind is that we may be sharing food utensils unwittingly. Do not take it for granted that the knife and the fork, the plate and the wine glass placed in front of you at a restaurant, or at a friend's house, are perfectly clean and sanitary. Always inspect utensils closely before using them, and never shy away from asking for a replacement if something doesn't look perfectly clean. Remember, if you can *see* dirt on the surface, just imagine how much more contamination is not visible to the naked eye.

When traveling, or trying out a new restaurant, I always make sure that I have a few alcohol wipes handy. Actually, it is a good idea to carry them all the time. They can make the difference between a pleasant dining experience or getting violently ill. So, even if that teaspoon looks clean, albeit a bit dull, or if that tiny spot on the plate looks fairly harmless to you, go to work with a disinfectant wipe before you eat.

Teach your children not to share eating utensils, cups, soda cans, drinking glasses or bottles with their friends. Make sure that they understand the dangers.

Never Share Personal Toiletry Items

These include combs, hairbrushes, razors, toothbrushes, roll-on deodorant, make-up and other personal hygiene products. Again, you are guaranteed to share, and share again, in an abundance of germs that another person has been collecting and spreading all over his or her toiletry items. Teach your children not to use other people's personal toiletry items. You should also avoid sharing eye drops, lip balm and contact lens cleaning supplies with other people.

BASIC RULES

Always Expect the Worst

Never assume an object or a surface is clean or germ-free. Unless absolutely sure, avoid it, don't touch it directly, or clean and disinfect it before handling, touching or using. If touching a potentially contaminated surface is unavoidable, always wash your hands immediately afterwards, using correct hand washing technique.

Never assume that other people are scrupulous about their hygiene or considerate towards others. Don't rely on others to protect you against germs. It is your responsibility, and yours alone, to prevent infection.

Protect Cuts, Scratches and Burns

This is especially important for the hands and forearms. Our skin does an excellent job protecting our bodies by keeping germs out. Very few disease-causing microorganisms are capable of entering directly through the skin. There are some exceptions, including hookworms and members of the papilloma virus genus that cause common skin warts.

Broken skin presents an unprotected gateway for harmful pathogens into the body. Touching a contaminated doorknob when the skin on your hand is perfectly healthy and unbroken is not the end of the world, provided that you refrain from touching your nose, eyes, mouth or genitals; and that you don't handle food before washing your hands. Healthy skin forms a solid barrier against germs. But even the smallest cut on the skin surface of your palm breaks that protective barrier. Bacteria, viruses, fungi and some parasites can enter the body freely.

There are three steps you should take to ensure that wounds do not become infected:

- **Clean** – Carefully clean the injured area. Use hot water and soap, and rinse to remove any dirt. If hot water and soap are not available, rinse the area thoroughly with clean cold water.
- **Disinfect** – Disinfect the area with alcohol, iodine, hydrogen peroxide, or one of the disinfectant solutions available from the pharmacy. Do not rinse with water again; let the disinfectant dry on the skin.
- **Protect** – There are two parts to protecting broken skin. First, we need to create a chemical barrier by applying an antimicrobial cream or lotion to the area. This serves the double purpose of killing any germs left in or around the broken skin and fighting off any germs that get into the area later. Second, we have to apply a physical barrier in the form of a plastic bandage ('band-aid') or other suitable wound dressing. This prevents dirt and germs from entering the broken skin. If this seems like overkill to you, bear in mind that we need to mimic the skin's ability to block out germs, and that is a tough act to follow.

There are also some convenient new products available on the market that combine plastic bandages with an antimicrobial agent. Some are infused with an antibiotic lotion and provide excellent protection against a wide range of bacteria. One of the new products I really like is a plastic bandage that uses silver in the wound pad. Silver acts as a natural antibacterial. Laboratory testing showed that silver reduces bacterial growth like *Staph. aureus, E. coli, E. hirae* and *Pseudomonas aeruginosa* in the dressing. Silver dressings are used regularly in hospitals to help control infections in major wounds and burns.

Other useful new products include spray-on or paint-on liquid bandages that dry rapidly on the skin to form a flexible, breathable and waterproof protective barrier. If bandages are unavailable, use a clean paper towel or tissue to cover the wound.

Be Prepared

At a minimum, always carry hand sanitizer gel, antibacterial wipes, extra strength facial tissues and plastic bandages with you. Add disinfecting spray or wipes if you travel or have to use public washrooms frequently. Pack water filters and purifiers if you travel to areas where drinking water is unsafe. Be aware of all infection hazards in your surroundings and take the necessary precautions to protect your health.

Carry your own sanitized items with you and avoid using public facilities. For example, carry your own pen to use at store checkouts or reading material for the doctor's waiting room. Avoid public water fountains; bring your own drinks. Before you use any public item, consider who else may have used it before you.

Isolate Those Germs

Keep sick family members separate from the rest of the household if possible. Re-arrange sleeping and eating arrangements if necessary. Don't send sick kids to school, day care or other activities. If at all possible, don't transport sick and healthy people in the same vehicle, and leave healthy kids at home when you go to the doctor's office, clinic or hospital.

Teachers should separate sick children and make arrangements for them to be picked up from school as soon as possible. Stay at home when you are sick. Sick employees should be sent home by management. If you are concerned about co-workers coming to work when they are sick, take it up with your manager or union representative. Don't hesitate to ask fellow employees to go home if they are ill, especially during flu season. Managers in any food service business should never allow sick employees to stay at work.

Disinfect the House

Use germ-killing cleaning products, bleach, steam or boiling water to regularly disinfect the house. Wipe down the phone, remote controls, computer keyboard and mouse, doorhandles, bathroom surfaces, toys, kitchen countertops and other frequently used surfaces. Wash dishes in the hottest water possible and allow to air dry, or use a dishwasher. Microwave dishcloths for 60 seconds to kill bacteria, or sanitize them in a household bleach solution.

BASIC RULES

This concludes the chapter on the basic precautions we can (and should!) take to avoid the germs that cause disease and infection. I urge you to make these basic precautions a routine part of your daily life. It will dramatically reduce your risk of contracting infectious diseases, and you and your family will be safer and healthier for it.

PUBLIC WASHROOMS

Public washrooms are notorious for harbouring and spreading the germs that cause infectious disease. And I am not referring exclusively to the visibly filthy and disgusting washrooms we find all too often these days. Even washrooms that appear sparkling clean on the surface can be contaminated with a frightening array of bacteria, viruses, fungi and parasites. Germs flourish in every nook and cranny of the average washroom, not only in the obvious places such as toilet bowls and urinals. A number of factors combine to make washrooms highly conducive to the survival and procreation of germs, and therefore very risky places for humans.

These risk factors include:

- high traffic;
- surfaces being touched by many hands in various states of contamination;
- the intended purpose of washrooms;
- damp or wet surface areas;
- the poor hygiene habits of many people; and
- inadequate cleaning and disinfecting of facilities.

PUBLIC WASHROOMS

Any surface in a public washroom that can be touched or brushed against is a potential breeding ground and staging area for germs.

A study of 25 public washrooms by the University of Arizona Microbiology Department showed that the most contaminated areas are the toilet floor, the sink and the taps, and high-touch objects such as toilet seats and handles. In another study of hotel bathrooms, it was found that toilet seats had lower levels of bacteria such as *staphylococci* than bathtubs, sinks and floors. This means that the area around the sink in the typical public washroom is one of the most contaminated parts of the facility, compared even to toilet bowls and urinals! Ironically, the very part of the washroom that we associate with cleaning and ridding our hands of germs, is where the biggest danger lurks. So even if you avoid the obvious and visible dangers, such as sitting directly on toilet seats or touching soiled surfaces, you are still very much at risk.

One of the main concerns in washrooms is fecal contamination. At least 100 different types of microbes occur in normal feces. There are many millions of bacteria in one gram of feces. The presence of *E. coli*, or other bacteria of the coliform bacilli group on a washroom surface is a tell-tale sign of fecal contamination.

In addition to *E. coli*, the following germs thrive in the average public washroom:

- *Salmonella* (typhoid)
- *Shigella* (bacillary dysentery)
- *Vibrios* (cholera)

SURVIVAL OF THE CLEANEST

- *Entamoeba histolytica* (amoebic dysentery)
- *Giardia lamblia* (giardiasis)
- *Enterobius vermicularis* (pinworm)
- Hepatitis A & E viruses (jaundice)
- Rotaviruses and other viruses that cause diarrhea
- Cold viruses
- Influenza viruses
- Respiratory syncytial virus (the most common cause of bronchiolitis and pneumonia)
- Chicken pox
- Measles
- Mumps
- Rubella
- Smallpox
- Scarlet fever
- Streptococcus bacteria (strep throat)

This chapter will help you understand and avoid the potential threats to your health when you use public toilet facilities. Armed with this knowledge, you and your family can safely navigate any washroom without fear of contracting an infectious disease. We also include guidelines and standards for clean and safe public washrooms. This is useful, even if you are not responsible for keeping a public washroom clean; it provides a benchmark against which you can evaluate the washrooms in your workplace, school, favourite restaurants, or any other public place you or your family frequently visit. Do not hesitate to bring any problems to the attention of the facility's management. Or better yet, give them a copy of this book. If you are responsible for managing or maintaining a public facility, you will find the practical information in this chapter useful.

Using Public Washrooms

The *first* golden rule for using public washrooms is: DON'T! Avoid using public washrooms as much as is humanly possible without damaging your health. Having made that statement, I will be the first to agree that it is not practical or comfortable, and often impossible to altogether avoid using public toilets. To completely avoid them means never leaving the house, and most of us don't want to do that. However, it is possible, by planning ahead and changing a few habits, to limit our use of public washrooms quite substantially. The following examples will illustrate what I mean.

Break the habit: I used to always go to the washroom in the cinema complex after the show. We live only ten minutes away! In most cases, waiting another ten or fifteen minutes to go to the bathroom makes no real difference. I realized that I was doing this as a matter of habit. Now I wait until I'm home, and that's one more visit to a public washroom avoided. If you plan to go for dinner after the movie, and you know that the washroom at your favourite restaurant is cleaner than the busy facilities at the cinema, wait until you get to the restaurant before you use the washroom.

SURVIVAL OF THE CLEANEST

Plan ahead: If you have a busy day of shopping and running errands scheduled, plan your route to include one or more stops at home. That will give you the chance to use your own bathroom and, as a bonus, you get a short break from your hectic day. Avoid drinking coffee, alcohol or other beverages that increase the frequency of washroom visits.

If you have to break rule one, always follow the **second** rule, which is to never touch any surface or object in a public washroom with your bare hands. Always use a paper towel or other suitable barrier to protect your hands when you:

- open or close faucets;
- raise or lower toilet seats;
- flush toilets;
- dispense soap;
- dispense paper towels;
- push the button on hot air dryers; and
- touch doorhandles.

The **third** rule is to always wash your hands *before* using the toilet. This is not a printing error. The first thing you should do before using any toilet, including at home, is to thoroughly wash your hands. You may think this doesn't make sense; we've always been told to wash our hands *after* using the bathroom. That remains true, of course, but we have not been told the whole story.

Consider the logic. We touch any number of surfaces and objects during the normal course of our day: doorknobs, money, telephones, keyboards, to name but a few.

PUBLIC WASHROOMS

We may shake somebody's hand or pet a dog. The skin on our hands, provided it is healthy and intact, does an excellent job protecting us from the germs we pick up this way. As long as we don't touch our noses, eyes or mouths, and remember to wash our hands before eating or handling food, this does not pose a serious threat to our health. But, if we don't wash our hands before using the toilet, we can transfer those germs onto our genitals. These parts of our bodies are highly vulnerable to infection, due to several factors: thinner and more sensitive skin, the presence of mucous membranes and the warm, moist conditions inside our underwear. Now you can see why we need to wash our hands *before* using the toilet.

Please refer to the section on keeping hands clean in the *Basic Rules* chapter for guidelines on how to safely wash your hands and avoid recontamination in public washrooms.

The *fourth* rule is: AVOID direct contact with the toilet seat. If you can manage it, squat a few inches above the toilet instead of sitting down. I realize this is not easy or possible for many people to do, but at least try and see how it goes.

If sitting down cannot be avoided, always cover the seat with a disposable seat cover (if available), paper towels or toilet paper. Very few facilities actually provide disposable seat covers. That is unfortunate, because it is a very effective and inexpensive precaution against the spread of germs. It just makes a lot of sense. Like antibacterial soap, I strongly feel that providing

SURVIVAL OF THE CLEANEST

toilet seat covers in public toilets should be compulsory. In the meantime, make a point of asking for them to be made available at the office, at restaurants, shopping malls, at your children's school or any places you or your family frequently visit. You have the right to a germ-free washroom at work, and if your regular restaurants want to keep you as their customer they should take your request seriously.

Whether you use a proper seat cover, or improvise with paper towels or toilet paper, always first wipe the surface of the seat carefully with toilet paper or paper towels. Use several paper towels, or roll off enough toilet paper to allow you to wipe the seat without your hands coming into contact with the surface. Be sure to remove any fluid or other visible matter. Be very careful not to touch any part of the toilet with your bare hands. Safely dispose of the soiled paper towel or toilet paper and flush the toilet. Cover the seat with the seat cover, paper towels or toilet paper. Drape several layers of toilet paper over the front rim of the toilet bowl. This will prevent any part of the genitals from coming into contact with the inside rim of the toilet.

Another option is to use a disinfectant spray or wipe to remove dirt and destroy germs on the toilet seat. There are several excellent products available on the market for this purpose.

Disinfecting wipes contain active ingredients like quaternary ammonium and alcohol. If used correctly they will kill most germs, including the bacteria commonly found in washrooms and the viruses that cause hepatitis and flu. Antibacterial wipes intended for personal use can also be used to disinfect toilet seats, although they may not be as effective against some viruses.

Disinfectant sprays are easy to use and are effective against a broad range of germs. They have powerful ingredients like ethyl alcohol, phenol (carbolic acid), hydrogen peroxide and quaternary ammonium that are effective against bacteria, viruses and fungi. Recommended surface contact times range from a few seconds to ten minutes. Always read and follow the instructions for use printed on the label.

Both wipes and sprays come in various packaging sizes that are convenient for travel or for keeping handy in a pocket, purse or backpack. A word of caution on disinfectant sprays: with the increased security at airports nowadays you will most likely not be allowed to take any kind of spray or aerosol container in your carry-on baggage or on your person. Take sufficient wipes instead.

To use disinfectant *spray* correctly, follow these steps:

- Flush the toilet. Keep the lid closed while flushing.
- Wipe the seat surface with paper towels or toilet paper.
- Spray a generous amount of disinfectant on the seat surface, and on any surfaces inside or outside the bowl that could come into contact with your skin. Men should pay attention to the inside front rim of the bowl.
- Leave on for the required surface contact time. This may vary depending on the product used.

SURVIVAL OF THE CLEANEST

- Wipe any excess disinfectant from the seat with clean paper towels or toilet paper.

When using disinfectant *wipes*, follow these steps:

- Flush the toilet. Keep the lid closed while flushing.
- Wipe the seat surface clean with paper towels or toilet paper.
- Thoroughly wipe the seat surface with a disinfectant wipe.
- Wipe any other surfaces that can come into contact with your skin.
- Leave the disinfectant on the seat surface for the minimum time recommended by the manufacturer, typically between 30 seconds and four minutes.
- Wipe any excess disinfectant from the seat with clean paper towels or toilet paper.
- Men should drape several layers of toilet paper over the front rim of the toilet bowl to keep their genitals from coming into contact with the inside rim.

Some situations warrant the use of a disinfectant *and* covering the seat. Use both when you have to use a toilet that is visibly dirty, when traveling or when using the toilet in a washroom with heavy traffic.

Rule *five:* Always close the lid before flushing the toilet. The spray caused by the flushing water spreads small, germ-laden droplets through the air that are deposited on your skin, clothes and washroom surfaces. You can also be infected by inhaling the airborne germs.

PUBLIC WASHROOMS

Rule number *six* goes without saying: wash your hands after using the toilet. Follow the steps described in *Basic Rules* for correctly washing your hands.

Rule *seven* concerns the purse, backpack, schoolbag and shopping bag dilemma. Do *not* place purses or bags on the counter next to a public washroom sink. Hang them on wall- or door-mounted hooks if available, sling them across your shoulder or ask a companion to hold them for you. Anything you put down on a washroom counter is guaranteed to pick up several nasty microbes. These germs get a free ride to wherever the bag or purse goes next. Anything that has been in contact with a washroom counter or floor should be disinfected without delay. Disinfectant wipes are well-suited to the task. They are convenient to use, effective and easy to keep handy in your car, office or in your purse.

It goes without saying that you should never place your purse or bag on the floor in a public washroom. Never.

The *eighth* rule is the one most often overlooked: Avoid recontamination. This is really unfortunate. Far too many people pay careful attention to all the other basic rules when using a public washroom, only to undo everything by directly touching the doorhandle on their way out. They may as well not have bothered. The bottom line is that public washrooms are high-risk, germ-infested places, and any surface you touch is potentially contaminated with a number of micro-organisms that can make you very sick, or even kill you. For detailed guidelines, please see *Basic Rules*.

In addition to protecting ourselves, following the basic rules for using public washrooms breaks the chain of infection. If you avoid contracting that stomach flu virus at the office, you don't pass it on to your family. The kids don't take it to school and your spouse doesn't infect his or her colleagues at work. You also set a good example for others to follow. As more and more people start to adopt smart washroom habits, the world becomes a safer and healthier place for us all.

Hygiene Standards for Public Washrooms

The following are the minimum acceptable standards for keeping public washrooms clean. Avoid using washrooms that don't meet these requirements and report them to the responsible persons or the appropriate authorities.

- Public washrooms should be cleaned and disinfected at least daily, more often in high-use facilities.
- Soap dispensers should be cleaned, disinfected and filled with antibacterial liquid soap daily.
- Paper towel dispensers should be clean, fully stocked and should function correctly.
- Toilets, toilet seats, urinals and urinal screens must be clean, dry and free of soils, urine and body fluids.
- Sinks should be clean, dry and free of any residues.
- Drain covers must be clean and free of litter, lint, mop strings, dirt, and other residues.

PUBLIC WASHROOMS

- All restroom floor surfaces must be clean, dry, slip resistant and free of soils, dirt and body fluids.
- Vents should be clean and free of lint and other residues. Fans should work.
- Mirrors and metal fixtures should be clean and free of smudges, finger marks, water spots, streaks, and other soils and residues.
- Restroom air must be fresh and free of unpleasant odours.
- Partitions, doors, doorknobs, walls, and ceilings must be clean and free of body fluids, smudges, finger marks and water spots.
- Countertops and ledges have to be clean, dry and free of any deposits.
- Lights should be working properly and light fixtures should be clean.
- Trash should be removed from the restroom at least daily and disposed of properly. Trash should be properly removed from all receptacles, and clean liners installed in the clean receptacles.
- Toilets and urinals should flush properly and not be blocked.

Access to clean, uncontaminated public washrooms is your right. Don't be afraid to speak up and insist on that right. Improving the sanitary conditions in one public washroom makes the world a healthier and safer place for many people.

FOOD SAFETY

Each year in the United States, approximately 76 million people get sick, 325,000 are hospitalized, and 5,000 die from foodborne illness. In Canada, several hundred deaths occur annually as a result of foodborne diseases. The US Centers for Disease Control and Prevention (CDC) estimates that about 70 percent of all cases of foodborne illness occur in food service operations; compared to 20 percent traced to homes. Food processors account for three percent. Most foodborne illnesses can be prevented by taking a few simple precautions. And yet, almost everyone has experienced a foodborne illness at some point.

Members of a typical North American household get their meals from a combination of sources: meals prepared at home from store-bought ingredients, restaurant or cafeteria meals, and take-out food from fast food outlets or delis. We also occasionally have dinner with friends or family at their homes, and sometimes prepare food in the outdoors when we go camping or backpacking. We have direct control over the safe handling and preparation of food when we prepare meals at home or at a campsite; we only have indirect control when we buy take-out meals, eat in a restaurant or school cafeteria, or have dinner at a friend's house. We directly ensure the safety of the meals we prepare at home by paying careful attention to the freshness and quality of the ingredients we purchase, by properly storing perishable items, and by following food safety guidelines for handling and preparing food.

We can indirectly control the safety and the quality of meals prepared by third parties by selecting only those restaurants, fast food outlets or delis with high food safety and hygiene standards, and by accepting dinner invitations only from those friends and family members who are meticulous about hygiene and food safety.

Food Safety at Home

It is a common myth that people only get sick from restaurant or take-out food. An estimated 20 percent of cases of foodborne illnesses occur when food is prepared at home. If food is handled and prepared safely, most of those can be avoided. All food may contain some natural bacteria, and improper handling gives the bacteria a chance to grow. Also, food can be contaminated with bacteria from other sources that can make you ill.

Illnesses caused by contaminated or unclean food can be very dangerous, especially to young children, older adults, pregnant women and people with weakened immune systems.

There are a number of steps you can take to prevent food contamination. The next section covers the Food Safety guidelines for buying, storing, handling, preparing and serving food at home.

SURVIVAL OF THE CLEANEST

Use Caution When Buying Food

- Buy your food only from stores with clean (pun intended) food safety records. Your local health department will keep a record of food safety violations, and some will have the information posted on their web sites. Avoid any stores with recent or serious violations.
- Avoid stores that look unclean, or where you observe unsafe handling or storage of food products. Pay special attention to areas where meat, seafood, dairy, poultry or eggs are displayed, handled or stored.
- Shop for groceries when you can take food home right away so that it does not spoil in a hot car. If this is not possible, or if you have a long drive home, or when shopping in hot weather, take a cooler box or bag in the car to keep perishable products from spoiling. Be sure to place a few ice bricks or a bag of ice inside to keep everything nice and cold. Some grocery stores sell insulated shopping bags that will keep food cold for shorter periods. They are great for keeping frozen products from thawing.
- Buy perishable food such as meat, seafood, eggs and dairy products last.
- Carefully inspect food products for freshness and look for any signs of contamination. Learn how to check meat, poultry and fish for freshness. Always check expiry dates on perishable products. Never buy any items that are past or close to their expiration dates. Allow for the time food products may sit in the

FOOD SAFETY

refrigerator at home before they are used. If you buy an item close to its expiry date, there is a good chance it will expire before you get time to eat it.
- Check packaged food for tears and canned goods for bulges or dents. Do not buy an item if the packaging is damaged or leaking.
- Don't let poultry, meat, seafood, eggs and dairy come into contact with other food, as they are most likely to contain bacteria.

Store Food Correctly

- Unpack food immediately when you get home.
- Wipe the outside of containers and food packaging with a disinfectant wipe, or use a clean paper towel moistened with disinfectant. Diluted chlorine bleach is an effective and inexpensive disinfectant. Avoid getting any disinfectant on the food.
- Refrigerate dairy products, eggs, raw meat, poultry, and seafood right away. Store separate or use containers to prevent contaminating other foods in the fridge. Store raw meat, poultry and seafood on a tray to prevent juices from dripping onto other food.
- Never store raw and ready-to-eat meats or seafood together in the refrigerator meat drawer. Pick one or the other and let everyone in the household know which type of meat should be stored in the drawer.
- Frozen food should be stored in the freezer without delay. Do not re-freeze frozen food that has started to thaw; use or discard it.

SURVIVAL OF THE CLEANEST

- Set refrigerators at 4° C/40° F and freezers at -18° C/0° F.
- Regularly clean and disinfect the refrigerator and freezer. Clean up any spills immediately and disinfect the area.
- Store dry foods (rice, flour, pasta, breakfast cereal) in airtight containers in a cool, dry place to protect against insects and rodents that can carry harmful bacteria.
- Store all food items away from cleaning products.
- Keep all food storage areas such as refrigerators and cupboards clean.

Prepare and Handle Food Correctly

- Thoroughly wash your hands before, during and after handling, preparing, cooking, and serving food. Wash your hands after handling raw meat, poultry, eggs or seafood. I strongly recommend using a good quality antibacterial liquid hand soap in the kitchen. Always follow the steps for correct hand washing as described in *Basic Rules*.
- Use disposable paper towels for drying your hands. Avoid using cloth towels in the kitchen.
- Clean and disinfect any kitchen surfaces, trays and cutting boards before, during and after preparing food. Use hot water and soap or a commercial cleaning product to thoroughly clean the areas. Apply disinfectant and let it stand for two minutes or longer, depending on the manufacturer's contact time

FOOD SAFETY

recommendations. This keeps the germs in contact with the disinfectant longer. Look for products that contain chlorine bleach. Chlorine or household bleach is a very effective disinfectant. To use chlorine bleach as a sanitizer, mix one teaspoon of bleach with a litre/quart of water and spray or wipe the bleach solution onto the area. Leave the bleach solution on the surface for at least two minutes. Then rinse and air dry. Follow the directions on cleaning product labels and always read safety precautions.

- Use paper towels to wipe up food spills and dispose of safely.
- Cloths used to clean and sanitize kitchen surfaces *must* be cleaned and disinfected often. Wash cloths and dry them in the dryer. Disinfect cloths in a strong chlorine bleach solution (three tablespoons per litre of water or about ¾ cup of bleach per gallon). Soak cloths in the solution for at least five minutes. Then rinse and hang them out to dry.
- Never use sponges for cleaning and sanitizing tasks. Bacteria multiply rapidly in a wet sponge containing food soil.
- Wear clean clothes or a clean apron and make sure there is no pet or human hair on your clothes.
- Any other people in the food preparation area should take the same precautions.
- Wash raw fruits and vegetables thoroughly under running water before eating or preparing them. This will not remove all micro-organisms, but it will reduce the number present. Germs have been found

SURVIVAL OF THE CLEANEST

on a variety of fresh produce, and outbreaks of foodborne illness have been associated with many types of produce. If the skin is contaminated, pathogens can move into the fruit when it is sliced. Removing the skin or rind reduces the risk of infection.

- Defrost frozen food on a plate either in the refrigerator or in a microwave, but not on the counter.
- Cook food immediately after defrosting.
- To prevent cross-contamination, always keep cooked and ready-to-eat foods separate from raw foods. Cross-contamination is the transfer of germs from raw food to ready-to-eat food. Use different dishes and utensils for raw foods and for cooked foods. When grilling outdoors, always use a clean plate for the cooked meat.
- Do not use one cutting board for all foods. Have at least two separate cutting boards: one for raw meat, seafood and poultry; and another one for cooked food, salads, fruit and other food that don't require cooking before eating. Non-porous cutting boards made of hard plastic are easier to clean than wooden cutting boards.
- Always follow the guidelines for properly cooking foods: Do not eat raw or partially cooked eggs. Avoid eating other foods that include raw or partially cooked eggs. Cook poultry until it has an internal temperature of 82° C/180° F. It is done when the juices run clear and it is white in the middle. Never eat rare poultry. Cook fish until it is opaque or white

FOOD SAFETY

and flaky. Cook ground meat to 74° C/165° F. It is done when it is brown inside. This is especially critical with hamburger meat.

- Limit hand contact with ready-to-eat foods by using single-use plastic gloves, tongs, paper towels or napkins.
- Because harmful bacteria grow at room temperature, keep hot food hot at 60° C/140° F or higher, and keep cold food cold at 4° C/40° F or cooler. This is especially important during picnics and buffets.
- Do not leave perishable foods out for more than two hours. Avoid leaving food out at all in hot weather.
- Promptly refrigerate or freeze leftovers in suitable containers or in plastic bags.
- When in doubt, throw it out. It is much cheaper to throw out bad food than it is to pay expensive medical bills or miss work.

Properly Clean and Disinfect Dishes

Whether you wash dishes in a dishwasher or by hand, always start with these steps:

- Wash your hands before handling dishes.
- Scrape off any leftover food and discard properly.
- Soak pots and pans in a hot water and dish detergent solution for 20 to 30 minutes before washing.
- Pre-soak cutlery in hot water for at least 15 minutes.
- Thoroughly rinse all dishes, cutlery, pots and pans before washing them.

SURVIVAL OF THE CLEANEST

Follow these steps when *washing dishes by hand*:

- Use separate sinks for washing and rinsing.
- Use clean dish brushes or cloths reserved for washing dishes. Do not use sponges. Sponges are ideal germ traps and incubators.
- Wash dishes in hot water and use a suitable dish detergent. Water should be at least 44° C/111° F. Hotter is better. Use rubber gloves to protect your hands from scalding.
- Change the water if it becomes visibly dirty, feels greasy or if the detergent stops foaming.
- Use proper brushes for glasses, cups and mugs.
- Rinse washed dishes in the second sink. Use clean, hot water with a minimum temperature of 44° C/111° F. If only one sink is available, remove washed dishes from the sink and place them on a clean, non-absorbent surface. Drain the sink, wash it thoroughly with hot water and dish detergent, rinse and fill with clean, hot water for rinsing dishes.
- Never use a towel to dry dishes. Air dry on a clean, non-absorbent surface or use a drying rack.
- Any dishes, cutting boards, cutlery, containers or appliances used to prepare or store raw meat, seafood, poultry, eggs or any other potentially hazardous foods should be sanitized. A solution of one teaspoon household bleach per litre of water (one tablespoon per gallon) makes a very effective and inexpensive sanitizer. Prepare sanitizing solution in a clean sink, or create an extra sink by placing a clean

plastic container on the counter. Fill it with the sanitizing solution and soak the utensils for five to ten minutes. Drain and air dry.

- Clean and sanitize dish brushes and cloths after each use. Launder dishcloths frequently and dry them in the dryer. This helps to kill germs. Brushes can be washed in the dishwasher. Dishcloths can be sanitized by heating the wet cloth in a microwave oven for one minute on the highest setting. Dishcloths and brushes can also be disinfected in a solution of three tablespoons of chlorine bleach per litre of water (¾ cup per gallon). Mix the solution in the sink or in a plastic container. Soak brushes and cloths in the solution for at least five minutes. Then rinse and air dry.

- Kitchen sinks, especially in and around the drains, were found to be some of the most germ-infested areas in North American homes. In one study of 15 household surfaces, the kitchen sink had the second highest germ count. Sinks should be washed with hot water and soap after each use and sanitized at least daily. A simple, inexpensive and highly effective remedy is to fill the sink with a solution of ¾ cup of household bleach for each gallon of water. Wait five to ten minutes before removing the plug. Do not rinse with water and allow to air dry. This will disinfect the sink and the drain hole and leave it germ- and odour-free.

Note: Sanitizing becomes more important if someone in the household is sick or at risk for foodborne illness due to a weakened or compromised immune system. All dishes and utensils used by sick or at-risk individuals must be sanitized.

Dishes and utensils washed in a *dishwasher* will have most pathogens removed by the strong mechanical action of the hot water and detergent. Hot water used in the rinsing cycle sanitizes the dishes. Using the heated drying cycle of the dishwasher further increases its effectiveness against germs. Additional chemical sanitizing of dishes and utensils is usually not necessary when a dishwasher is used.

Dishwashers have to be used and maintained correctly to ensure that each load of dishes is perfectly cleaned and disinfected. Improper use and maintenance of the dishwasher can cause illness in the household.

To use the dishwasher correctly:

- Follow the manufacturer's instructions.
- Clean scrap trays and wash ports before each use.
- Group dishes by size and shape.
- Place dishes to allow water to reach the entire surface of each dish. Do not overload the dishwasher.
- Place bowls, cups, mugs and glasses with their bottoms up.
- Place cutlery in a proper cutlery basket or tray.
- Mix cutlery to prevent spoons or forks nesting inside one another.
- Use the correct kind of detergent for your type of dishwasher.

FOOD SAFETY

- Hot water (at least 60° C/140° F) should be used for the wash cycle.
- Water temperature for the rinse cycle should be at least 82° C/180° F.
- Always use the heated drying cycle.
- Ensure that the dishwasher maintains the required time for each cycle.
- If water is not heated to the minimum temperature required for each cycle, or if a heated drying cycle is not available, dishes may not be fully sanitized. In this case always disinfect any dishes and utensils used to prepare or store raw meat, seafood, poultry, eggs or other hazardous foods. Prepare a solution of one teaspoon household bleach per litre of water (one tablespoon per gallon) in a clean sink. Soak utensils for five to ten minutes. Drain and air dry.

To maintain the dishwasher correctly:

- Ensure that it is in good working condition.
- Always follow the manufacturer's instructions for using and maintaining your dishwasher.
- Contact the manufacturer or service agent if you need additional information or advice.
- All repairs should be done by a qualified technician.
- Rinse jets and clean wash ports regularly to prevent clogging.
- Remove debris after each use.
- Scrub and disinfect the inside of the dishwasher at least twice a week.

- Leave the door open when it's not in use. This allows the inside to dry and air out, and prevents mold and odours from developing.
- Check water temperatures frequently. If there is no digital read-out on the outside, or if it's not working, get a service technician to check the temperature. You can also buy a maximum registering dishwasher thermometer that measures water temperature during washing and rinsing, and holds the highest temperature reading until the thermometer is shaken.

Single-use temperature tags or indicator strips are also available. Tags are attached to a plate or other utensil and change colour if the required temperature is reached at the utensil surface. Indicator strips are more sophisticated and will measure a range of up to five temperature levels.

Restaurants, Cafeterias and Take-out Food

We cannot control how food is handled and prepared in restaurants, school cafeterias or fast food kitchens. Some people blindly trust that food safety rules are meticulously followed everywhere; while other, more philosophical folks, believe it's the luck of the draw whether you get sick or not.

Neither approach is healthy. We may not be able to completely eliminate our chances of buying a contaminated meal, but we can take several steps to reduce our risk. These steps include understanding food safety risks, doing our homework, being able to identify the danger signs, and exercising caution when choosing the places we buy meals from. By following the practical guidelines provided below, you can dramatically reduce the risk of eating a contaminated meal.

Although restaurants are just one link in the food-supply chain, their role in preventing foodborne illness is crucial. We would like to believe that every manager in the restaurant and fast food industry is obsessive about food safety and hygiene; that all their staff are properly trained and supervised; that only healthy individuals are allowed to work in the kitchen; and that they take every possible precaution to serve safe food. We assume they all understand that the cost of implementing health and safety precautions is much less than the damage a single outbreak of foodborne illness can cause to their business. That it is better to be safe than sorry. Don't count on it. It is human nature to cut corners and to think nothing bad will happen. Examples of illness caused by contaminated food abound, ranging from serving a single meal that makes a diner sick, to large outbreaks like the Jack-in-the-Box tragedy a few years ago.

Most countries have health and safety regulations and standards in place for food service operations. Standards do however vary widely from country to country, and can even differ from one region, or city, to another within one country. Outbreaks of foodborne illness occur even in countries like Canada or Switzerland with exceptionally high and uniform standards. We simply cannot rely on every single staff member, in every single restaurant or fast food outlet, to do everything correctly all of the time. The world doesn't work that way. You do need to take steps and have the knowledge to mitigate your risk as much as possible. It is your responsibility to protect your health and that of your family.

In many developing countries, food safety and hygiene standards, or any form of regulation, are virtually non-existent. You need to take a number of additional precautions to protect your health when traveling in these countries. These steps are described in detail in the *Travel* chapter.

Understand the Risks

The same threats to food safety present in the home are found in restaurant and fast food kitchens – at exponentially increased levels! The number of kitchen staff, the variety of meals prepared and ingredients used, the rush to get orders out the door, use of high-volume food processing equipment, and more exposed surface areas all contribute to increase the risk of contamination. The presence of large quantities of dirty dishes also poses a major health risk if not handled properly.

Foodborne illnesses in food service establishments are caused by eating food that has been contaminated. The contaminants may be biological (bacteria, viruses, fungi and parasites), chemical (cleaning supplies, pesticides, and food additives), or physical (dirt, broken glass and crockery that accidentally get into food). Contaminants often get into food through careless behaviour and ignorance on the part of kitchen staff.

FOOD SAFETY

Harmful substances or germs can be introduced into food service operations and transferred to food in a number of ways:

- contaminated food ingredients;
- unsanitary equipment;
- supplies;
- customers;
- dirty utensils;
- dishcloths;
- human hands; and
- contact between raw food and ready-to-eat foods.

The most common foodborne illnesses are caused by *Salmonella, Campylobacter,* Calicivirus or Norwalk-like virus, *Shigella* and *E. coli.* Other diseases that can propagate via contaminated food include infections caused by the hepatitis A virus, and the *Giardia lamblia* and *Cryptosporidium* parasites.

Salmonella bacteria can make people sick with a disease called salmonellosis. Symptoms can include diarrhea, abdominal cramps, vomiting and fever. Symptoms typically appear six to 48 hours after infection and can last for several days. Foods that are most likely to carry *Salmonella* bacteria include raw and undercooked meats (especially poultry), raw milk, eggs and sprouts. Fruits and vegetables can become contaminated with *Salmonella* bacteria if they have been exposed to contaminated soil, or have come in contact with a contaminated product or surface, such as a countertop or hands.

SURVIVAL OF THE CLEANEST

Campylobacter bacteria cause fever, diarrhea, and abdominal cramps. It is the most commonly identified bacterial cause of diarrheal illness in the world. These bacteria live in the intestines of healthy birds, and most raw poultry meat has *Campylobacter* in it. Eating undercooked chicken, or other food that has been contaminated with juices dripping from raw chicken is the most frequent source of this infection.

Shigella bacteria mainly occur in the intestinal tract of humans. It is rarely found in other animals. It gets into food through human contamination and poor hygiene by food service staff. People can also be infected by drinking contaminated water, such as water supplies polluted by untreated sewage. The consumption of *Shigella*-contaminated food or water, or contact with infected people may lead to shigellosis, more commonly known as dysentery. Symptoms include diarrhea, abdominal pain, fever, vomiting and dehydration. The most common foods to carry *Shigella* are salads (potato, shrimp, tuna, chicken, macaroni, fruit and lettuce). Turkey, rice, beans, desserts, strawberries, spinach, raw oysters, luncheon meats and milk may also carry *Shigella*.

E. coli 0157:H7 bacteria live in the intestines of cattle, poultry and other animals. When an animal is butchered, the bacteria can be transferred to the meat's surface. Ground beef can be contaminated because the grinding process distributes surface bacteria throughout the meat. If the meat is not thoroughly cooked throughout, some bacteria can survive. Illness can occur after ingesting only small amounts of *E. coli 0157:H7* bacteria. It can also be spread by contact with an infected person or by contaminated surfaces. Symptoms may include flu-like symptoms, diarrhea, abdominal pain, vomiting and fever. It can cause a type of kidney failure and blood disorder called Haemolytic Uremic Syndrome (HUS). *E. coli 0157:H7* bacteria have also been found in raw and undercooked meats, cheese, lettuce, unpasteurized milk, raw fish, cream pies, mashed potatoes and other prepared foods.

Calicivirus, also known as Norwalk-like virus, is an extremely common cause of foodborne illness. It causes acute gastrointestinal illness, usually with more vomiting than diarrhea, that resolves within a few days. Unlike some foodborne pathogens that have animal reservoirs, it is believed that Norwalk-like viruses spread primarily from one infected person to another. Infected kitchen workers can contaminate food as they prepare it.

The *hepatitis A* virus is spread primarily through food or water contaminated by feces from an infected person. Hepatitis is a liver disease with symptoms that include jaundice (yellowing of the skin and eyes), fatigue, abdominal pain, loss of appetite, nausea, vomiting, diarrhea, low grade fever and headache. It can be fatal, with an average of three deaths in every 1,000 cases.

Do Your Homework

Before buying food from any restaurant or fast food outlet, find out if they have a record of food safety violations. Contact your local health department for the information. Many authorities make the information available on their web sites as well. It's also a good idea to ask friends or co-workers if they are aware of any food safety problems at the food service outlet you plan to visit. Avoid any places with serious or recent violations and absolutely avoid places with multiple violations on their record.

Become fully familiar with the principles of food safety. Reading this book will arm you and your family with all the knowledge you need to understand and avoid the causes of foodborne illness in food service operations. If you study and follow the practical advice and guidelines provided in this book, you can dramatically reduce the risk of becoming seriously ill from eating a contaminated meal from a restaurant, fast food outlet or any other food service operation.

Since I started applying these principles more than ten years ago, I have not had a single foodborne illness. During this period I've eaten at countless restaurants and I have traveled extensively, including a number of trips to developing countries with less than stellar food safety records. Foodborne illness can, and should be, avoided.

Recognize the Danger Signs

Take a quick walk through the dining or service area to see if it's clean and tidy. Things to take notice of include an excessive number of uncleared tables, a dirty or sticky floor, soiled or grimy tables and countertops, and unpleasant odours. Pay attention to the appearance of the servers: are they neat; are they wearing clean outfits;

do any of them display any cold, flu or other symptoms; and do any of them have any uncovered cuts, sores or burns? If the public area of a restaurant or fast food outlet is visibly dirty or messy, just imagine what else lurks hidden from your view. Think about all the invisible germs that thrive in filthy conditions. Avoid any food service outlet with litter inside or outside the premises.

In countries like Canada and the USA, food service outlets have to display operating permits as proof that they comply with the standards and regulations set by health authorities. Also look for food safety training certificates or certificates awarded for food safety excellence programs.

Take a look at the kitchen. If the kitchen isn't visible from the dining or service area, request to see it. If they refuse, walk away. Sometimes you'll be told that health regulations prohibit members of the public in the kitchen area. This is a valid excuse in many cases, but you do not have to take 'no' for an answer. Explain that you do not need to go inside the kitchen area and that you only want to take a quick look from the kitchen doorway. You don't need a close-up or lengthy inspection to spot problems in a restaurant kitchen.

If a kitchen is obviously dirty and disorganized, with dirty dishes stacked to the ceiling, garbage bins overflowing, and people running around frantically, you are at risk of being served contaminated food. Go somewhere else for your meal.

Remember to report what you saw to the appropriate health authority as soon as possible. It only takes a few

SURVIVAL OF THE CLEANEST

minutes to send an e-mail that can prevent an outbreak of disease and potentially save somebody's life.

Even if a kitchen looks reasonably clean at first glance, there are other danger signs to look for. Pay attention to the appearance of kitchen staff. Look for the following:

- Are they clean?
- Are they wearing clean uniforms or aprons?
- Do any of them appear to be sick (sneezing, coughing or sweating excessively)?
- Do any of them have open cuts or burns?
- Are their hands clean?
- Are they wearing clean latex or plastic gloves?
- Are their fingernails short and clean?
- Is anybody wearing nail polish or false finger nails?
- Are they all wearing hair restraints?
- Is anybody wearing jewellery?
- Do they all seem to know what they are doing?
- Are they disorganized?
- Is anybody picking or blowing his nose, scratching his face, touching his mouth or rubbing his eyes?
- Is anybody eating or smoking?

The presence or absence of sufficient hand washing stations is another critical factor. Kitchen staff will not wash their hands frequently if it is difficult or inconvenient for them to do so. A proper hand washing facility should have a wall-mounted sink, hot water tap, liquid soap dispenser and paper towel dispenser or hot air dryer.

FOOD SAFETY

Take a look at how raw meat, fish and poultry are handled. These foods should be kept separate from other foods to avoid cross-contamination.

Do you see any leftover food returned from the dining room? Leftovers should be disposed of in the garbage immediately and shouldn't be left out in the food preparation area. A pile of dirty dishes in or near the food preparation area is another warning sign.

Look for proper garbage disposal facilities. Garbage bins should be a safe distance from food preparation and storage areas; they should have proper linings and should not be overflowing with garbage. There should be no foul or rotten odours coming from the garbage disposal or any other area in the kitchen.

Pay careful attention to the condition of the floor and countertops. Keeping the floor and work surfaces clean is a very elementary part of kitchen hygiene. If this is overlooked, you can bet your bottom dollar that other safeguards are being ignored.

If all of this sounds like a comprehensive health and safety inspection to you, don't despair. With a little practice, and after you've done it a couple of times, it takes no more than a few minutes to scan a kitchen to get a general impression and pick out any non-compliance with food safety principles. It may well be the best few minutes you've ever invested in your health.

Before you sit down or order, inspect the washroom. If there are members of either sex present in your party, check out both washrooms. The state of the washrooms is an excellent barometer for the general standards of hygiene,

SURVIVAL OF THE CLEANEST

cleanliness and safety in any food service establishment. It is also a truly universal yardstick; a filthy restaurant washroom in New York is equally indicative of other potential health risks as a filthy washroom anywhere else in the world. No place can ever be cleaner or safer than the condition of its washrooms alludes to. An impeccably clean, tidy, properly ventilated and well-supplied washroom, though not an unqualified guarantee, is usually a good indication that the place is well-managed and that high standards of hygiene and cleanliness apply in other areas as well.

Carefully inspect the table when you sit down in a restaurant. In take-out premises, examine the order and pick-up counters, condiment shelves, pop dispensers and litter receptacles. These areas should be perfectly clean and free of any spills and grime. Pay special attention to salt and pepper shakers, condiment bottles and any other dispensers on the table, or on the condiment shelves. Greasy, sticky dispensers and menus, covered in smudges; or condiment bottles smeared with product residue on the outside are indicators that no attention is paid to the details of keeping everything clean. If the details are overlooked, the chance of finding unsafe conditions increases substantially.

In addition to alerting us to the presence of other potential health hazards, these objects are germ traps in their own right. If you have handled any of them during your inspection, avoid touching your nose, eyes or mouth and wash your hands as soon as possible and before you eat anything. Use sanitizer gel or wipes to disinfect your hands if washing isn't practical.

FOOD SAFETY

Examine drinks or food brought to your table. Thoroughly inspect plates, glasses, cups and cutlery for any dirt, grime, smudges or fingerprints. Teaspoons are excellent indicators of the general state of hygiene in a food service outlet. If they can't keep their teaspoons clean, chances are that other good hygiene and food safety practices are falling by the wayside. Never eat at a place with dirty teaspoons.

If any food item on your plate, or any drink you are served does not smell, look or taste right; send it back immediately. Never assume that it is fine, or that you are imagining things. Pay special attention to meat, seafood, poultry, and dishes made with cream and eggs. These foods will often have a noticeable odour when spoiled.

The platinum rule is: *When in doubt, don't eat it!*

Should your server refuse to take the meal back, or insist that there is nothing wrong with it, get up and leave, even if it means paying for a meal you didn't eat. It is a lot cheaper, and much less painful, to pay for something you didn't get to eat, than it is to get sick. The average cost of a restaurant meal is a lot less than most people earn in a few hours at work, hours you stand to lose if you are sick. The same rule applies to take-out food. Throw it away if it doesn't seem right. If at all possible, take the food back to the outlet or inform them via phone or e-mail that your meal was spoiled or contaminated. They are most likely unaware of the problem and can take steps to prevent more contaminated meals being sold if they are informed. Your actions can prevent other people from getting sick, or save someone's life.

SURVIVAL OF THE CLEANEST

Important note: If you or any member of your family get sick after eating restaurant or take-out food, or any other store-bought or packaged food, immediately report the incident to the appropriate health authority. Deliver the suspect food to the designated office or laboratory as soon as possible. If you are unable to do so right away, double-bag the food in heavy-duty plastic bags and store it in the back of the fridge, taking care to avoid contact with other food items.

CLEARLY MARK THE BAG: DO NOT EAT! CONTAMINATED FOOD SAMPLE.

Inform everyone in your household about the sample and make sure they all understand the danger. Store it out of reach of small children. Alternatively, place the sealed sample in a small cooler box with an ice brick or sufficient ice to keep it cold until you can deliver it to the health authority laboratory or office. Wash your hands thoroughly after handling the contaminated food.

Don't be afraid to speak out for fear of offending or upsetting restaurant staff. Most food service owners, managers, kitchen staff and servers are sincere and bona fide in their efforts to serve safe and uncontaminated food. In many cases, they are simply not aware of food safety hazards that are present in their operation. This could be due to ignorance, or being inundated with other operational issues. By pointing out hygiene and food safety trouble spots, you are doing them a favour and helping them to improve their business. It is safe to assume that no restaurant owner wants to be responsible for an outbreak of a potentially deadly foodborne illness, and

FOOD SAFETY

that they will accept, if not appreciate, your polite and constructive comment. A rude or defensive reaction is an indication of the wrong attitude towards food safety (and customer service!) Take your business elsewhere. For good measure, report the incident to the local health inspector. You and your family have the right to safe, uncontaminated food. Food service operators should respect that right.

Limit the number of food service outlets you buy meals from. It is simply a matter of odds. The more places you eat at, the greater your risk of getting sick. It's like driving too fast: the more times you speed, the higher your chances are for getting a ticket or having an accident. On the flip side, the longer you eat at one place without ill effect, the less your chances are of being served a bad meal.

Always have a few single-use alcohol wipes handy. Use these to wipe cutlery, the rims of glasses and cups, the table surface around your plate and armrests.

Never share food or utensils with other people at your table. Not even with family members. In the first place, he or she could be infected with a cold or flu virus, or any number of harmful viruses and bacteria. Sharing food and utensils means sharing saliva, and germs thrive in saliva. There is another, less obvious, reason not to share food or utensils. If one member of the party is served a contaminated meal, sharing food will spread the germs to others too. It is bad enough if one person around the table gets sick. Sharing puts everybody at risk. The same goes for sharing drinks; it's not a wise thing to do. Teach your children not to share food with their friends.

Be polite to your server. Never insult or treat your server in a rude manner. It is not uncommon for upset food service staff to tamper with customers' food before serving it. Video footage abound of restaurant staff caught on hidden surveillance cameras spitting or urinating on food. There are recorded cases of feces, blood, or even semen being intentionally introduced into food. In other cases, pieces of glass, metal and food waste were added to food. So, in addition to being polite because it is the right thing to do, you avoid the possibility of getting some really nasty stuff in your food. It goes without saying that you should never insult the chef!

A Final Word on Food Safety

Applying the principles explained in this chapter has protected me from foodborne illness for over ten years. I am confident that I will not contract a foodborne disease during the next ten years and beyond either, because I intend to continue following the rules for eating out safely. They work, and they can work for you too.

Camping

In addition to the guidelines for safely handling and preparing food at home, more precautions are necessary when you prepare food at a campsite or in the backcountry. Food safety in the outdoors is addressed in the *Camping & Outdoors* chapter.

MOTOR VEHICLES

Our cars are catchment areas for all the germs we accumulate on a day-to-day basis. Most of us spend many hours a week behind the wheel or in the passenger seat. This gives us ample opportunity to deposit germs on, and to pick up germs from, everything we touch inside the car. Whatever we do, or wherever we go, chances are we'll end up in the car several times on any given day. And all the germs we come into contact with during our errands are transferred onto the steering wheel, doorhandles, gear shift, cup holders, and everything else we touch in the car. Some germs can survive for hours, even days on any of these surfaces. This means our vehicles also serve as germ exchanges; anyone traveling in the car can be infected.

Always keep your car clean and germ-free. At a minimum, regularly clean and disinfect all frequently touched surfaces in the vehicle. Start with obvious areas, like the steering wheel, gear shift, parking brake, radio dials, power window switches and doorhandles. Disinfectant wipes do an excellent job of cleaning and disinfecting in one step. Buy the larger, heavy duty kind. It is a good idea to keep a container with wipes in the vehicle. Some brands come in round plastic dispensers

SURVIVAL OF THE CLEANEST

that will fit in a cup holder. This makes it easy, and serves as a reminder, to disinfect high-risk surfaces often. Wipes work fine for sanitizing hands and for many other cleaning tasks in the vehicle.

It is a good practice to keep the interior of your vehicle clean and litter-free. Dust, grime and litter provide microbe-friendly habitats where harmful germs can grow and spread very quickly. Never leave food wrappers or drink containers lying around inside the vehicle. You might as well place a sign in the rear window that says 'germ heaven inside.' Clean up any food or drink spills as soon as possible. Bad odours in the car should be investigated to determine and remove the cause.

Regularly vacuum carpets and upholstery to remove dust and other debris that provide a sanctuary for germs. Use an aerosol air cleaner that contains ethyl alcohol or phenol to reduce airborne bacteria, viruses and fungi in your vehicle.

Keeping your vehicle clean is just as important when you are on a road trip.

PUBLIC TRANSPORTATION

All forms of public transportation are high-risk areas for contracting infectious diseases. Buses, trains, subways and taxis all provide perfect breeding grounds and distribution systems for germs. They contain all the risk elements for contamination. They form bottleneck areas with high human traffic, and have several exposed surfaces touched by many different hands during any given period of time. Even if you are fortunate enough to live in a city with very high standards of cleanliness for its public transportation facilities and equipment, do not let your guard down. They may look perfectly clean, but the interiors of most forms of public transportation harbour high levels of harmful micro-organisms. Remember, germs cannot be seen with the naked eye, and may be present even on brightly polished surfaces.

   I am most definitely not suggesting that we all stop using public transportation. Using public transportation is one of the few viable options we have available to reduce traffic congestion and pollution in our cities. If anything, people should be encouraged to use public transportation more often. Fortunately, by being aware of the dangers we face, and by taking a few common sense precautions, it is possible to safely commute to the office and elsewhere. This chapter provides you with the knowledge to protect yourself against infection when using urban public transportation.

The Dangers

We'll use the average city bus or school bus as an example to illustrate the health hazards found on all forms of public transportation. The risk of infection on a bus comes from four sources:

- **High traffic** – the sheer number of people who pass through the average city bus on any given day is a major source of germs.
- **Infrequent cleaning and disinfecting** – most city buses run pretty much around the clock and they are not properly cleaned on a daily basis, let alone disinfected.
- **Increased surface contact** – surface areas in a bus are touched by many hands in varying states of cleanliness, leaving behind a frightening array of germs.
- **Litter** – people often leave food wrappers and drink containers behind on the bus. These items contain food residue and traces of saliva, which are perfect carriers and incubators for germs. Used hypodermic needles and other drug-related detritus are sometimes left behind on city buses or subways, and pose severe health and life-threatening risks. A single jab with a contaminated needle can infect you with deadly viruses like hepatitis or even HIV, the virus that causes AIDS.

PUBLIC TRANSPORTATION

The Precautions

There are a number of basic precautions you can take to safeguard yourself when using public transportation. We'll continue using the example of a city bus, although these rules apply to any form of public transportation.

- Avoid touching anything with your bare hands.
- Carefully inspect the area before you sit down. Look for things like food spills, drink containers, food wrappers or, heaven forbid, blood or other body fluids. Always scrutinize the seat and floor for hypodermic needles, any drug use paraphernalia or sharp objects. If you find a needle or other sharp object, move away from the area and immediately inform the driver. Warn other passengers to stay clear of the area.
- Avoid sitting close to other people if possible. This greatly reduces your chances of contracting colds, flu or other contagious infections they may have.
- Never eat, drink or handle food when you are traveling on a bus.
- Be careful not to touch your eyes, nose or mouth when traveling on a bus or until you've had a chance to wash your hands. Touching your eyes, nose or mouth in an unhygienic environment like a bus is a sure-fire way of becoming infected.
- Always carry hand sanitizer or disinfectant wipes. Clean your hands as soon as you sit down, and before handling any personal items like a laptop, cell phone, reading glasses, etc.

SURVIVAL OF THE CLEANEST

- Consider wearing disposable latex or plastic gloves if you frequently travel by bus and can't avoid touching handrails, support straps or other objects. You should definitely wear gloves if you have any condition that compromises the integrity of the skin on your hands.
- Wash your hands as soon as you can after completing your journey. Do not eat or handle food before washing your hands and use the correct washing technique described in *Basic Rules*.
- Consider wearing disposable face masks during flu season or any other time there is an outbreak of an infectious disease. The face mask will only protect you from airborne germs; remember to wash and disinfect your hands more often during flu season.

There are a number of things we can do to make public transportation safer and more pleasant for everybody:

- Report any unsanitary or unsafe conditions to the transit authority. If issues are not resolved within a reasonable time frame, do not hesitate to go higher up the bureaucratic and political chain of command.
- Engage the media to create awareness of public transport-related health and safety problems and the corrective actions required to fix them. The media can also play a very important role to promote more considerate behaviour and better hygiene among passengers.
- Encourage your friends, relatives and especially your children to be more aware of the dangers and to be more vigilant when using public transportation.

PUBLIC TRANSPORTATION

By protecting ourselves we make using the bus, train or subway a safer, less stressful experience, and are therefore more likely to use public transportation. By making a contribution towards cleaner and safer conditions in general, we help encourage others to leave the car at home and use public transportation.

WORKPLACE HYGIENE

Most provinces, states and other jurisdictions have regulations and programs in place to promote health and safety in the workplace, and to protect workers against occupational hazards. It is outside the scope of this book to cover the entire field of occupational health and safety. This chapter focuses on the basic requirements for a clean and germ-free work environment, and the steps you can take to protect your health at work.

You have the right to a clean and safe work environment. Compare your workplace to the benchmark facilities and standards described in this chapter. How does it measure up? If your workplace doesn't have the required facilities, or meet all of the standards, do something about it. Request additional facilities, or ask for existing facilities to be upgraded. Insist on clear rules and policies for hygiene in your work environment. This needn't be a confrontational process. A polite, constructive approach usually works best. Having a clean workplace and healthy workforce is in the employer's best interest as well. Follow the chain of command as far as possible; involve your immediate supervisor or manager first. In a unionized workplace, involve your shop steward or union representative.

WORKPLACE HYGIENE

The following facilities, services and policies should be in place and available at your place of work:

- Daily professional cleaning of all work areas, washrooms, lunch rooms, kitchens, meeting rooms and other high-traffic areas.
- Daily garbage removal.
- Sufficient washroom facilities that meet the hygiene standards detailed in the chapter dealing with *Public Washrooms*. Employers should also install touchless faucets and paper towel dispensers, and provide antibacterial soap, disposable toilet seat covers and disinfectant wipes. It is a good idea to install a dispenser for hand sanitizer by the door *outside* the washroom so people can disinfect their hands without the risk of recontamination.
- Service or equipment to regularly clean and disinfect telephones, keyboards, computer mice, machine consoles and any other equipment that see a lot of hand traffic. At a very minimum, disinfectant spray or wipes must be available near workstations and easily accessible to everyone.
- Clean, properly equipped lunch room and kitchen facilities. There should be sufficient refrigerator space and a dishwasher or proper sink to accommodate the number of employees who use the lunch room. Refrigerators and dishwashers should be cleaned regularly and properly maintained. Signs or posters with food safety rules should be displayed in the lunch room and kitchen. Local health authorities can provide useful posters or pamphlets.

SURVIVAL OF THE CLEANEST

- Clean, fresh and purified drinking water.
- Hand sanitizer or disinfectant wipes in meeting rooms, training rooms, washrooms, lunch rooms and kitchen areas, reception areas and any other high-use areas.
- A strictly enforced policy that makes it mandatory for employees to stay home when they are sick with or recovering from any infectious type of disease; for example, a cold, flu, Norwalk virus, hepatitis A, meningitis or infectious diarrhea caused by a virus or bacteria. Managers and supervisors should have the authority to send sick employees home.

You also have a responsibility to protect your own health, and to help make the workplace cleaner and healthier for everyone. There are several steps you can take to avoid contracting infections or spreading germs in the workplace:

- Follow all the basic precautions for avoiding infection described in *Basic Rules*.
- Follow the rules for using *Public Washrooms*.
- Be food safe when you eat at work. See *Food Safety*.
- Set a good example. Share your knowledge on the topic of preventing infection with your co-workers. Lend them your copy, or better still, buy them a copy (or several copies) of this book.
- If you are sick, stay home. If you are a manager or supervisor, send sick employees home.
- Report any unsanitary conditions to the appropriate people in your organization.

WORKPLACE HYGIENE

- Keep your own workspace clean and germ-free. A study sponsored by the Clorox Company found that the average desk harbours 20,961 germs per square inch – 400 times more than the average toilet!
- Wash the coffee maker pot when it's your turn to make coffee. Use dish washing detergent and hot water to thoroughly clean the inside and the outside, including the handle and lid. When pouring a cup of coffee at other times, use a paper towel to protect your hand. Coffee maker pots are very effective germ exchanges, and most people don't give them a second thought. Consider for a moment the coffee maker at your workplace. How many different people handle the pot every day? Are all those hands perfectly clean and germ-free? Chances are they are not. Besides, it only takes one unwashed hand to contaminate the handle. As an added bonus to the germs, coffee makers provide a warm, often wet environment – pathogen paradise. I strongly recommend using disposable paper filters in the coffee maker. Re-usable filters should be washed each time a fresh pot is made.
- Protect your hand with a paper towel when operating the water cooler spigot. Like the coffee maker, it is a high-traffic, high-risk area. For information on cleaning and maintaining water coolers, please see the *Drinking Water* chapter.
- If your desk also serves as your lunch table, use disinfecting wipes before and after lunch to reduce bacteria and other germs on your desk.

PUBLIC TELEPHONES, ABMs & SHARED COMPUTERS

The telephone, automated banking machines (ABMs) and computers are three of the most important inventions of our age. Very few of us can imagine what life would be like without any one of these technologies. We take them for granted. Unfortunately, we also often overlook the fact that they are ideally positioned to spread infectious disease.

I am not suggesting that you avoid public telephones and ABMs altogether, nor am I saying you should steer clear of Internet cafés on your next overseas vacation. However, you should be aware of the risks and should be extremely cautious when using these facilities. Contracting a serious infectious disease from a contaminated telephone, ABM or computer keyboard is a very real and present danger.

Public Telephones

It's a scary list: cold and flu viruses, feces, saliva, viruses that cause respiratory problems, and bacteria that cause

PUBLIC TELEPHONES, ABMs & SHARED COMPUTERS

dysentery and other deadly infections. It would be bad enough if the list referred to a badly neglected public washroom. Actually, these are contaminants and germs that regularly show up on public telephones!

A single public telephone can be used by hundreds of people every day in a busy street, mall or airport. The law of averages dictates that some of them must be sick; some would have been in contact with sick people; and most will have some level of germ contamination on their hands.

Telephones spread infectious disease in two ways: First, germs are transmitted via the telephone mouthpiece. When a person with a respiratory illness talks, coughs, or sneezes, tiny droplets of moisture (called fomites) spray from their mouths, carrying bacteria or viruses into the air. If a sick person is talking into a telephone, fomites land on the mouthpiece and remain there. When the next person uses the telephone, the moisture containing the infectious germs is still present on the mouthpiece, with his or her mouth and nose only millimetres away. Speaking into the mouthpiece creates airflow that dislodges the germs, causing them to become airborne. Occasionally people will accidentally touch the mouthpiece with their lips, providing another way for the bacteria or viruses to enter their bodies.

The second way telephones transmit disease is via the handle. Bacteria, viruses and fungi on people's hands are transferred to the telephone handle when they make a call. When other people use the phone they get the germs on their hands. If they neglect to wash their hands and eat, handle food, or touch their eyes, noses or mouths, infection can occur. The transfer of disease by hands is very common when using high-traffic transfer points like public telephones and doorhandles.

Public telephones are very rarely cleaned, if ever. Even if they were, they're only as hygienic as the last person who made a call.

The guidelines below provide a practical way for safely using public telephones. They apply to all shared telephones, such as those in the workplace and even at home.

- Avoid using public telephones. Use public phones for emergency or essential calls only. Wait until you are home to make social calls. Consider getting a cellular phone.
- Avoid heavily used telephones. Look for a phone in a quiet part of the shopping mall or airport; walk a block or two away if you are on a busy street.
- Assume that any telephone is contaminated with germs and a source of infection. Public telephones should be approached like guns: always assume they are loaded.
- Sanitize the handset with a disinfectant wipe or spray. Using a disinfectant can dramatically reduce the level of germs and therefore reduce your chances of infection. If you don't have disinfectant wipes or spray handy, use a paper towel, napkin or facial tissue to hold the handset.
- Cover your dialing finger with a paper towel, napkin, facial tissue or any piece of paper or plastic.

PUBLIC TELEPHONES, ABMs & SHARED COMPUTERS

- Avoid touching the mouthpiece with your lips, and keep the earpiece a few millimetres away from your ear.
- Don't eat, drink or touch your face while using a public phone.
- Wash or disinfect your hands after using a public telephone.

Automated Banking Machines (ABMs)

Several studies show that ABM keypads harbour more germs than public restroom doorknobs. It's not really surprising. Many people touch them; the banks never seem to clean them; and more hands that touch a public washroom doorknob have just been washed, compared to the hands that touch the ABM. Tests show that ABM keypads can be contaminated with dangerous organisms like *strep A,* the microbe that causes flesh-eating disease and strep throat; *E. coli; Staph. aureus;* and other fecal-borne microbes that can cause dysentery and various serious infections. Scientists agree that the presence of bacteria like *E. coli* on ABMs poses a public health threat.

The following steps will eliminate most of the infection risks when using an ABM:

- Limit your use of ABMs as much as possible. Use credit or debit cards instead of cash. Plan ahead: Withdraw enough money for the next week or two instead of making several cash withdrawals. It will

SURVIVAL OF THE CLEANEST

also save you time and banking fees. Combine transactions to cut down on the number of visits to the ABM. If you are paid by cheque, ask your employer to directly deposit your salary into your bank account. Use Internet banking for bill payments and transfers.

- Always assume that the ABM keypad and screen are contaminated with dangerous pathogens and treat it as such.
- Do not touch the keypad directly. Protect your finger with a piece of paper or plastic, or use a disposable object to touch the keys. Disposable coffee stirrers work well.
- Never touch your face after using an ABM.
- Never lick the deposit envelopes! They have been handled several times in the process of unpacking and stocking the ABMs. Also, the glue on envelope flaps is not exactly manufactured to meet food-grade standards. Just tuck the flap inside the envelope to prevent money or cheques from falling out. If anything falls out, the bank will sort it out; it can't go further than the ABM's deposit compartment. Fortunately, some banks have started introducing self-sealing ABM envelopes. Hopefully all banks will soon follow suit.
- Disinfect your hands with hand sanitizer gel or wipes immediately after using an ABM. (You do remember not to leave home without enough sanitizer, don't you?) Wash your hands as soon as you can.

■ Do not eat or handle food until you have washed or sanitized your hands.

The same dangers and precautions apply to vending machines, ticket dispensers and the handheld payment devices used at restaurants and stores.

Shared Computers

Infectious germs can survive on computer keyboards and mice, making it easy for infections to spread to other users. In a study conducted at the Northwestern Memorial Hospital in Chicago, three bacteria commonly found in hospitals were deposited on keyboards and keyboard covers to see how long they could survive. Researchers typed on the keyboards to see if the bacteria could be transferred to the fingers. Two of the bacteria could survive for up to 24 hours on keyboards or keyboard covers. The third survived for up to one hour on the keyboard, long enough to infect other people. They found that the bacteria were easily transferred to fingers. Contamination increased relative to how often people used the keyboards.

In high-traffic areas like Internet cafés, the risk of spreading germs to others increases exponentially. The problem becomes even worse if equipment is not regularly cleaned and disinfected. The facts apply to any scenario where computers are shared by several people; for example, libraries, schools, Internet cafés and the workplace. Computer use everywhere is increasing rapidly. We need to be aware that all keyboards, mice,

SURVIVAL OF THE CLEANEST

printers, headsets, and other computer peripherals can be repositories and transfer points for infectious germs.

When using a shared computer, always follow these common sense guidelines:

- Assume that the keyboard, mouse, headset, and other peripherals are contaminated.
- Be considerate to the next user, and do not assume the previous user was as considerate as you are.
- Don't eat, handle food or touch your face while using a shared computer.
- Avoid touching your eyes, nose and mouth while using a shared computer.
- Always wash your hands before and after using the computer. Use a hand sanitizer gel or wipe if soap and water are not immediately available.
- If you share a computer with other persons, wipe the keyboard, mouse, headset, microphone, game controller, etc. with a moist disinfectant wipe before and after you use them. Do not get liquid between the keyboard keys, inside the mouse, or in any openings.
- Computer keyboards, mice and other peripherals in schools, Internet cafés, the office and libraries should be disinfected often to prevent the spread of harmful bacteria. Some disinfectant solutions need to remain on the surface for up to ten minutes to be effective.

SHOPPING

Stores are high-risk places for germ contamination, because of high human traffic, the fact that all items and people are funneled through the same checkout points, and because most stores never clean and disinfect their shopping carts and baskets. Food and grocery stores also harbour foodborne pathogens due to the presence of raw and perishable foods.

Most of us cannot avoid shopping altogether, nor can we expect that every single store will see the light and do everything possible to protect their customers from infectious diseases. It is up to us to be aware of the dangers posed by germs when we shop, and to take all the necessary precautions to keep ourselves and our families safe from infection.

This chapter will help you understand and avoid the potential threats to your health when shopping. Armed with this knowledge you and your family can enjoy shopping without contracting an infectious disease.

Shopping Carts and Baskets

The biggest danger of germ contamination for most shoppers is when they touch a shopping cart or basket handle. We touch them two or three times a week, and so do thousands of other people. It is not surprising that studies show shopping carts and baskets can spread germs. They are no different from doorhandles, washroom faucets, telephones, elevator buttons and other frequently touched objects. Whatever germs people have on their hands are left behind when they touch a shopping cart handle. One study in the USA found more bacteria on shopping carts than in public toilets. Supermarkets very rarely clean their shopping carts or baskets, if ever. How many times have you touched a sticky or grimy handle, or found litter, dirt and debris in a shopping cart?

Several studies found shopping cart and basket handles to be contaminated with blood, mucus, saliva, urine, fecal matter and a frightening array of bacteria and viruses, including *Staph. aureus, Enterococcus faecalis, Streptococcus pneumoniae, E. coli 0157:H7*, rotavirus, and hepatitis A. Infection with the *E. coli 0157:H7* bacteria can cause the often deadly disease Haemolytic Uremic Syndrome (HUS). The HUS disease attacks the kidneys, heart and brain.

Unsanitary shopping carts represent a health hazard, especially for our children and people with weakened immune systems. Dangerous bacteria can find their way onto a shopping cart and to shoppers who touch it.

In grocery stores, raw meat, seafood and poultry are major sources for the bacteria that find their way onto shopping carts or baskets. Between June 1999 and July 2000, researchers from the Department of Nutrition and Food Science at the University of Maryland sampled 825 packages of raw meat from 59 supermarkets in the Greater Washington, DC area. The meat in 179 of the packages sampled contained *E. coli* bacteria, 159 samples contained *Campylobacter,* and 25 contained *Salmonella*. These germs can easily migrate onto the outside of packaging when juices leak from the trays. Shoppers usually handle several trays of fresh meat, seafood or poultry in making their selections and transfer germs to shopping carts or basket handles. These germs can stay alive on the contaminated surfaces for hours or even days.

There is also reason for concern that carts are not sanitized after homeless people have used them to store and transport their possessions. In November 2001, television station KRON-4 conducted random tests of shopping carts recovered from homeless people in San Francisco. They tested several carts and found that half of them tested positive for *fecal coliform* bacteria, as well as *fecal strep* and *E. coli*. Incredibly, they found that when these carts were returned to the supermarkets they were immediately put back into service without being cleaned or disinfected.

The supermarket industry generally considers the risk of infectious germs on shopping carts and baskets to be very low and nobody is acknowledging that there is a problem. It is reasonable to assume that the cost of cleaning and disinfecting carts and baskets plays a role in shaping their point of view.

Yet, there are inexpensive and effective ways to sanitize carts and baskets and protect shoppers from harmful germs. A few progressive grocery store chains have implemented hand sanitizing facilities at cart corrals inside store entrances, and at meat and seafood counters. They provide instant hand sanitizing wipes to shoppers at these points to kill germs on their hands. The wipes can also be used to clean cart handles.

Some stores provide hand sanitizer gel or sanitizing wipe dispensers at various points throughout the store. Smaller food stores should consider attaching hand sanitizer dispensers to shopping carts.

For a number of years now, a cart sanitizing system has been available to supermarkets. It works like a miniature car wash and costs just a few pennies per cart to operate. To date, only two supermarkets have tested the system, and to the best of my knowledge it has not yet been implemented anywhere.

Even a simple intervention like wiping or spraying cart handles with a disinfectant once a day would go a long way towards protecting shoppers from infectious diseases.

Supermarkets should accept responsibility to protect their customers from infectious germs spread via shopping carts and baskets. Clean carts prevent illness and can save lives. Insist on your right to shop without risking your health or exposing your children to serious diseases. Hopefully one day supermarkets will pay heed and provide shoppers with a safe and healthy environment to shop in. In the meantime, take all the necessary precautions to protect yourself and your family from the potentially deadly germs on shopping carts and baskets. This chapter is your family's complete guide to germ-free and healthy shopping.

SHOPPING

Checkout Counters

All roads in the store lead to the checkout counter. Everyone and everything that leave the store pass through this checkpoint, and millions upon millions of germs with them. Checkout counters are as contaminated, sometimes more so, as shopping carts. If it weren't for the fact that, in most stores, checkouts are occasionally cleaned and disinfected, they would easily win the contest for the most contaminated surface in the store.

Food and other grocery items pick up a toxic cocktail of germs from the checkout conveyor belt and transfer these disease-causing microbes to your hands, kitchen counters and food storage areas. *E. coli* is once again the big culprit: there are regular reports in the news of *E. coli* infections that can be traced back to grocery store checkout counters.

Fellow Shoppers

Germs thrive wherever large numbers of people share limited real estate. Stores are no different. If anything, stores are a lot more contaminated. In addition to just crowding the area, people handle, touch or taste the merchandise; share shopping carts; and handle raw foods. In winter, the average large department store becomes an overheated biosphere filled with flu and cold viruses.

The way most large stores are laid out also contributes to the problem. Aisles are organized to maximize your exposure to all the merchandise in the store and to boost impulse buying. Ever notice how meat and dairy counters are always at the back of the store? Want bread and vegetables? Try the opposite end of the store. This ensures you have to walk through the entire store just to pick up a few basic food items. It also means a lot of people are spreading bacteria from the meat and dairy counters all over the place.

In-store pharmacies are also typically located in the back or off to one side. It is not unreasonable to assume that a fair percentage of people filling prescriptions suffer from some kind of medical condition. The law of averages dictates that at least some of them will have a contagious illness. The net result? Scores of contagious people wandering through the food aisles to pick up their medication.

But the worst is yet to come. A Minneapolis-based company started opening drop-in medical clinics *inside* Wal-Mart stores! The clinics are staffed by nurse practitioners who can diagnose and treat common ailments, such as flu, bronchitis and pink eye, and provide basic services, such as vaccinations. Apparently, part of the plan is to give patients pagers so that these potentially contagious people can walk around the store, doing their shopping while waiting for their appointments, and spreading germs all over the store.

Store Employees

In this day and age of people working multiple low-wage jobs to make ends meet, weak or non-existent union protection, and dwindling benefits, many people

SHOPPING

simply cannot afford to take sick days. The result is increased exposure to infectious germs for customers and co-workers alike, creating an ever-expanding chain of infection.

In addition, staff hygiene standards and policies in most grocery stores are simply inadequate to reduce the risk of infection for shoppers. There are no hand washing stations near checkout counters or in display areas that can be easily accessed by all staff. Inexpensive, logical solutions such as providing hand sanitizer to checkout staff are widely ignored.

Add in all the germs store employees pick up from money and payment cards, raw food items and dirty cash register keys, and you end up with a group of individuals who are extremely likely to accumulate and pass on germs.

Safe Shopping

Understanding where in-store infectious germs lurk enables you to take sensible precautions when you shop. While you cannot avoid or eliminate all the germs you encounter during shopping, the following steps will effectively reduce your exposure to germs and will help limit the spread of germs to your fellow shoppers and store employees. These precautions will make shopping a lot safer for you and your children. Safe shopping habits should be second nature for the entire family.

- Shop during off-peak hours or in smaller, less-crowded stores.

SURVIVAL OF THE CLEANEST

- Never go shopping without hand sanitizer gel *and* sanitizing wipes. Use both often and freely.
- Use sanitizing wipes to clean shopping cart handles and any part of the cart that will come in contact with your hands or your children's hands.
- Use sanitizing wipes in the meat department to remove meat juice from your hands.
- Use disposable shopping cart seat covers to protect small children against germs on the shopping cart. Choose products that cover the handle and other areas that children touch most often. Throw away or recycle used covers; don't re-use. Covers also protect others from your children's germs and diaper leaks.
- Avoid make-up testers. Studies show that testers are often contaminated with *Staphylococcus aureus* and *E. coli* bacteria, and the germs that cause pink eye and herpes.
- Carry your own pen to use at store checkouts.
- Keep your hands away from your face.
- Never eat or open any food items in the store or in the car on your way home, before you have had a chance to wash your hands.
- Avoid grocery store washrooms.
- Use caution when buying food:
  - Buy your food only from stores with clean (pun intended) food safety records. Your local health department will keep a record of food safety violations, and some will have the information posted on their web sites. Avoid any stores with recent or serious violations.

SHOPPING

- Use caution when buying food (continued)
    - Avoid stores that look unclean, or where you observe any unsafe handling or storage of food products. Pay special attention to areas where meat, seafood, dairy, poultry or eggs are displayed, handled or stored.
    - Buy perishable food such as meat, seafood, eggs and dairy products last.
    - Check packaged food for tears and canned goods for bulges or dents. Do not buy an item if the packaging is damaged or leaking.
    - Don't let poultry, meat, seafood, eggs and dairy products come into contact with other food, as they are most likely to contain bacteria. Place each item in a separate plastic bag.
    - Pay attention to how staff at deli counters handle food and report any unsafe practices to the store management.
    - Beware of food samples offered during in-store promotions. Samples are often left out for hours and can become contaminated by other shoppers' hands. Never try any samples that contain chicken, seafood, dairy or undercooked red meat.

MEDICAL FACILITIES

Doctors' Offices and Clinics

We associate a visit to the doctor with getting better. What most people don't realize, is that a visit to the doctor can be very hazardous to their health. As a rule, most people who visit a doctor or clinic suffer from one or more ailments. Generally, a fair portion of people in the waiting room will be sick from an infectious disease; many will be symptomatic. In flu season, the number of contagious patients climb exponentially. In other words, we share a lot of harmful germs in doctors' waiting rooms, surgeries and clinics.

So what are we to do? It is obviously not possible to avoid visiting the doctor altogether. Even those people blessed with perfect health sometimes have to consult with a doctor; or visit a clinic for preventive procedures like vaccinations, treatment of minor injuries or routine medical checkups.

We face multiple threats in the waiting room: a high concentration of airborne viruses, especially in flu season; and surfaces contaminated with sick people's germs. We are also typically exposed to a wide variety of germs in the waiting room.

MEDICAL FACILITIES

Visiting the doctor or clinic is a classic good news/bad news scenario. The bad news is that you cannot entirely eliminate the risk of contracting an infectious disease at the doctor's office or clinic. The good news is that by taking a few common sense precautions, you can dramatically reduce your exposure to infectious germs. By following the guidelines below, you can make your next visit to the doctor a much safer and less stressful experience for you and your family.

Precautions

- Avoid unnecessary visits to the doctor or clinic. If you only need to renew a prescription or get test results, do so by phone if possible. Otherwise you may end up with a more serious illness contracted in the waiting room. If you are taking a sick family member or friend to see the doctor, don't accompany them into the waiting room or surgery. Wait outside in the car or go for a walk. Unless of course it's a small child or a person who requires assistance, in which case you have to stay with them.
- Make appointments for early in the morning. Always try to get the first appointment on your doctor's schedule. That way you virtually eliminate spending time in the waiting room, there are typically fewer people around, and your doctor has not yet accumulated germs from other patients. Surgeries and clinics are typically cleaned and sanitized overnight, which means germ levels are generally lower early in the day. So get there early!

SURVIVAL OF THE CLEANEST

- Try to find a practice or clinic that has separate 'sick' and 'well' waiting areas. There aren't too many of those, unfortunately, and only the large practices have sufficient space for this type of arrangement. Hopefully, separate waiting areas is a growing trend and I look forward to seeing more of them. Separate 'sick' and 'well' rooms should be properly labeled, and staff should enforce compliance among patients.

   An exciting new concept does away with the waiting room entirely. A number of progressive practices in the United States have decided the best approach is to not have a waiting room at all, or to minimize its use by ushering patients to examination rooms as soon as they check in. Some offices have multiple examination rooms with doors that open directly to a parking lot. Patients can wait in the safety of their cars until it's their turn to see the doctor. Sadly, it will probably be a long time before all medical practices adopt this approach. Getting rid of the waiting room represents a major and potentially expensive change in how a medical practice operates. For most practices, implementation would require additional examination rooms, fewer appointments or both.

- Limit the time spent in the waiting room. Do not show up too early for your appointment; phone to check if the doctor is on schedule. If he or she is running late, delay your departure to arrive closer to the actual time of your examination. After checking in at the reception desk, wait outside the offices or in your car. If you cannot wait close to the waiting room,

MEDICAL FACILITIES

leave your cell phone number at the desk and have them call you when the doctor is ready to see you. Whatever you do, don't spend one minute more in the waiting room than you absolutely have to.

- Avoid surgeries or clinics without separate play areas for children. Sick children are like unguided missiles armed with biological warheads. They are prone to all kinds of infections, and they lack the awareness and social skills to avoid infecting others.

- Keep your children away from all toys, books, crayons and activity centres in the waiting room play area. To avoid the spread of germs, these things should probably be disinfected every five minutes. I doubt that many are even disinfected daily. Bring your child's favourite toy or book and ensure that other kids stay away from it. Remember to disinfect the toy when you get home.

- Don't go near the magazines and books in waiting rooms. Everyone who touches them leaves germs behind on the pages. Take your own book or magazine if you anticipate a long wait.

- Remember that everything in a doctor's office is a potential source of germs, including doorknobs, chair armrests, washrooms and even the pen and check-in register. Keep antibacterial wipes or sanitizer gel handy to clean and disinfect your hands. Sanitize children's hands more frequently.

- NEVER eat or drink in the waiting room. Don't allow your children to eat in the waiting room.

SURVIVAL OF THE CLEANEST

- Don't touch your nose, eyes, mouth or any other part of your body.
- Avoid sitting near a child or adult who is coughing or sneezing.
- Hold babies and small children or keep them in a car seat or stroller in the waiting room to minimize the number of surfaces and toys that they touch.
- Consider wearing disposable face masks during flu season or any other time there is an increased incidence of infectious disease in your community. The face mask will help protect you from airborne germs in the waiting room. Be sure to check if there are high-efficiency particulate-arresting (HEPA) filters installed in the ventilation and air conditioning ducts of the surgery or clinic. HEPA filters effectively remove airborne viruses and other germs. While they reduce some of the risk of infection from airborne pathogens, HEPA filters won't protect you from the germ spray if somebody sneezes or vomits two feet away from you, so you always have to exercise caution.
- Cover any cuts, burns or other areas of damaged skin, especially on the hands or arms prior to visiting the doctor or clinic.
- When you get home, scrub your hands, take a shower and wash your clothes on the hot cycle. Disinfect anything you wore or carried with you during the doctor's appointment: watch, purse, wallet, book, cell phone, kids' toys, etc. This may sound like a huge

task, but it takes only a few well-invested minutes. Be sure to use a broad-spectrum disinfectant that also kills other germs like viruses and fungi, not just bacteria. Disinfectant sprays or wipes that contain ethyl alcohol, phenol (carbolic acid), hydrogen peroxide or quaternary ammonium are effective against a wide range of germs.

- Remember that your doctor is exposed to many different infectious germs in a typical day. You don't have to treat him or her like a leper, but you cannot ignore the reality that your doctor can make you sick. Several research studies found stethoscopes, pens and white coats to be infested with harmful germs. One study even identified doctors' neckties as collecting areas and transfer points for pathogens. In an ideal world, all physicians are able to keep their clothing and hands perfectly clean and germ-free. I know I don't live in a perfect world, so I always assume the worst. Disinfect your hands and don't eat or handle food until you've had a chance to thoroughly wash your hands after being examined by a physician. Change your clothes and take a shower as soon as you get home.

Hospitals

More people in North America die every year from hospital-acquired infections than from auto accidents and homicides combined. About two million infections are acquired in US hospitals each year, resulting in over

SURVIVAL OF THE CLEANEST

90,000 deaths. An estimated 250,000 Canadians become sick and 8,000 die from infections contracted in hospitals each year. Those who survive often endure lengthy hospital stays and suffer long-term health problems.

Hospitals are filled with patients who are susceptible to infection due to their weakened immunity. Surgery, needles, and catheters can introduce germs into the body. Hospital staff often fail to take all the necessary steps to stop the spread of infection. The situation has become more dangerous because of the emergence of bacteria that are resistant to commonly prescribed antibiotics. Because these infections don't respond to treatment with antibiotics, the bacteria are referred to as 'superbugs.' Patients infected with superbugs can double their hospital stay: first recovering from the illness that brought them to hospital, and then recovering from the secondary infection. Patients admitted to hospitals generally expect that their stay will make them healthier, yet a growing number of patients are leaving the hospital with a serious infection.

Common hospital-acquired infections include:

- Methicillin-resistant *Staphylococcus aureus* (MRSA), a bacterial staph infection that causes abscesses, boils, severe pneumonia and blood poisoning. MRSA bacteria are resistant to the antibiotic methicillin.
- *Streptococcus pneumoniae* or strep, a fast-spreading 'superbug' that causes meningitis, sinusitis, ear infections and pneumonia.
- *Clostridium difficile* bacteria produce toxins that cause diarrhea and damage the cells lining the bowel. It can

cause critical illness and death in elderly or sick patients, or people with immune disorders.
- Necrotizing fasciitis, or 'flesh-eating disease,' is a strep infection.
- *Pseudomonas aeruginosa* causes pneumonia, urinary tract infections and bloodstream infections.
- ESBL-producing bacteria. Extended spectrum beta lactamase are enzymes that are resistant to antibiotics like penicillin. ESBL enzymes are most commonly produced by two bacteria: *E. coli* and *Klebsiella pneumoniae*; but can also be produced by other bacteria like *Salmonella, Proteus, Morganella, Enterobacter, Citrobacter, Serratia* and *Pseudomonas.*
- Vancomycin-resistant *Enterococci*, (VRE) is a bacterial infection that is resistant to the common antibiotic vancomycin.

The SARS infections in the Toronto area in 2003 were the result of hospital outbreaks.

High-risk Transfer Points

Hands

In-hospital infections are a major health problem, and dirty hands and fingernails are often responsible. It has been estimated that doctors, nurses and other hospital workers don't wash their hands properly 70 percent of the time. Discomfort is one reason for that failure. Certain antibacterial soaps and alcohol-based rinses can cause dryness and skin irritation.

SURVIVAL OF THE CLEANEST

It is your responsibility to ensure that the people who treat you, feed you and care for you in hospital have clean hands. It is your right as a patient not to be infected because of a caregiver's lack of hygiene. Insist that anyone who touches you, serves you food or administers medication, first wash and disinfect their hands. If you don't see them do so, politely ask if they have. It is a good idea to keep a bottle of alcohol-based hand sanitizer by your bedside and ask that hospital staff use it before attending to you.

Healthcare workers attending to you should also be wearing latex or vinyl gloves. The gloves not only protect them from contracting infections, but also reduce the infection risk for patients. Gloves should be changed between different procedures and before going to the next patient.

And don't forget to keep your own hands clean. Thoroughly wash your hands with soap and hot water when possible, especially after going to the bathroom and before eating. Use hand sanitizer if washing with soap and water is not practical.

Hospital Food

Hospital food has a well-deserved reputation for tasting bland at best. Many people do not realize that it can actually kill you, or at the very least, make you seriously ill. Think I'm exaggerating? Consider the following facts: Hospital food is prepared and served in an environment that is potentially much more contaminated with germs than typical food service operations. There are more airborne germs due to the concentration of a large number of sick people in one building. Even the best ventilation and air filtration systems cannot clean all the viruses and bacteria from the air all the time; some will end up on food or food preparation surfaces before they can be removed. Germs are also spread by food service staff who share washrooms and other facilities with nurses and other healthcare staff, and by hospital staff who move freely between the kitchen and patient wards. Preparing and serving large quantities of food virtually around the clock also increase the risk of contamination. It is ironic that so many expensive studies are being conducted to trace the sources of hospital infections, yet food, one of the most obvious culprits, is all but ignored.

There really is no safe way to consume hospital food. Your best bet is to avoid it altogether. Ask a friend or relative, one you know to be diligent about food safety, to bring in your meals during your hospital stay. Use your own utensils; eating safe food from a contaminated hospital plate voids your other precautions. The same holds true for water. Bring your own bottled water and ask visitors to replenish your supply. Drink only juice that is served in a sealed container. Don't allow hospital staff to open drink containers for you; they mean well, but you don't want to ingest the contaminants that may well be on their hands.

Visitors

People who visit friends and family in hospital mean well, and most patients appreciate the moral support and interest in their well-being. Unfortunately, hospital patients typically suffer from conditions that make them more susceptible to infection. This means that otherwise harmless germs on the hands of a visitor can cause serious illness if transferred to a recovering patient.

Most people would agree that receiving no visitors, especially during lengthy stays in the hospital, is not an option. We cannot ignore the dangers, however, and have to exercise caution and use our common sense.

The guidelines below will make hospital visits safer:

- Limit visitors to immediate family and close friends.
- Insist that people with flu or other infectious illnesses stay away.
- Ask visitors to leave small children at home.
- Exercise caution when eating candy and other snacks brought by visitors. Don't eat anything made with meat, seafood or dairy. Wash or peel fruit.
- Ask that visitors wash or disinfect their hands before spending time with you. Keep hand sanitizer gel by your bedside for visitors to use.
- If your insurance covers the cost of a private room, or if you can afford to pay for one, make use of it. That way you avoid fellow patients and their visitors.

Washrooms

Hospital washrooms are high-risk places for contracting infectious diseases. Don't use them unless you have to. Always exercise extreme caution when using a hospital

MEDICAL FACILITIES

washroom and take all the precautions described in the chapter on *Public Washrooms*.

Before taking a shower in a hospital bathroom, let the hot water run on full setting for two minutes. Wait for all the water on the shower floor to drain away before stepping in. This will reduce the germs that thrive in showerheads and on damp shower floors. I strongly recommend using a spray disinfectant to sanitize the faucets, showerhead and shower cubicle.

Computer Keyboards

Infectious germs, including drug-resistant bacteria, can survive on computer keyboards for as long as 24 hours. A study carried out at Northwestern Memorial Hospital in Chicago found that keyboards can contaminate a doctor's or nurse's hands, who could then infect patients. Computers are being used increasingly in hospitals. Some are installing computers in every ward and room.

Three types of bacteria are commonly found on computer keyboards in hospitals: Vancomycin-resistant *Enterococci* (VRE), methicillin-resistant *Staphylococcus aureus* (MRSA) and *Pseudomonas aeruginosa*.

Staph infections can cause skin rashes, boils and blisters, toxic shock syndrome and several other types of infections; *Enterococci* can cause abdominal infections, skin infections and bloodstream infections; and *Pseudomonas aeruginosa* can cause pneumonia and urinary tract infections.

Doctors and nurses normally wash their hands before attending to patients, but hand washing before or after using a computer is mostly overlooked. Most hospital staff are simply not aware of the problem.

As always, your best protection is to confirm that any healthcare workers attending to you have washed or sanitized their hands.

Water Faucets

A study conducted at the Ulm University Hospital in Germany found that stagnant water in hospital faucets is a major source of infectious germs in hospitals. They found that in 40 percent of cases of recorded bacterial infections, the faucet was the source. Hospital staff don't regularly clean taps in bathrooms and kitchens. Bacteria levels can build up quickly in the moist environment inside taps, especially in infrequently used taps.

Never drink tap water in a hospital!

Additional Precautions

There are a number of additional precautions that can help reduce your risk of hospital infections:

- Exercise caution.
- Question any conditions, procedure or activity that you are not comfortable with. Communicate your concerns in a respectful manner.
- Be vigilant about the quality of care you receive.
- Be aware of the catheter. Approximately 40 percent of hospital-acquired infections involve the urinary tract. The risk of those infections increases significantly if a

urinary catheter is left in place for more than two days. If you're still using the same catheter 48 hours after surgery, find out whether removal has been overlooked. If you start feeling urinary discomfort, the catheter may be clogged.
- Start moving as soon as you can. This can help prevent bedsores, another cause of hospital-acquired infections, as well as dangerous blood clots.

RECREATIONAL FACILITIES

Germs at the Gym

Working out at the gym is a way of life for many people. There is no doubt that exercise is good for us. It is a great way to stay in shape and strengthen the body. It boosts our immune systems, reduces stress and helps us sleep better. It may even slow down the aging process. Some people also enjoy the social interaction. However, gyms are also important links in the chain of communicable diseases.

Consider the following before your next workout:

- Researchers regularly find *E. coli* and *streptococcus* bacteria, flu viruses and fungi in gyms and on workout equipment.
- Many people contract athlete's foot (*tinea pedis*) at the gym. The symptoms of this fungal skin infection include cracked and blistered skin, itching and burning. Nails can also become infected by fungi living on shower and locker room floors. Symptoms include discoloured and brittle nails. Fungal infections are very difficult to cure and some people may experience recurring outbreaks for years.

RECREATIONAL FACILITIES

- The virus that causes plantar warts, papilloma virus, is often found in gyms. These warts grow on the bottom of the feet.
- The US Centers for Disease Control and Prevention (CDC) recently reported that methicillin-resistant *Staphylococcus aureus* (MRSA) bacteria may spread in recreational training facilities. MRSA is a major cause of hospital-acquired infections, is very difficult to treat and can have deadly consequences.

You may be picking up something else in addition to those weights. Dirt and germs on a person's hands, clothes, skin or shoes can be passed on to the next person who uses the equipment.

Take the following precautions to prevent infection at the gym:

- The first step to protect yourself is to disinfect the equipment before use. Many gyms will provide some kind of sanitizing spray, but I recommend taking your own disinfectant wipes or spray. That way you can be sure that it will be effective.
- Use hand sanitizer gel or antibacterial wipes to kill germs and clean your hands as you move from one piece of equipment to the next.
- Thoroughly wash your hands after using gym equipment, free weights and exercise balls. Be careful not to recontaminate your hands after washing, and follow up with hand sanitizer.
- Bring your own towels to place over gym equipment. Launder them after each workout session.

SURVIVAL OF THE CLEANEST

- Wear shower shoes or flip-flops in the shower and locker room to protect your feet from fungal infections. Never go barefoot in the gym.
- Change your socks and gym shoes immediately after exercising. Launder socks after each workout session and wash gym shoes occasionally in the hot water cycle. Sweaty socks and shoes are prime breeding grounds for fungi and odour-causing bacteria.
- Wash and dry your feet thoroughly after working out. Apply antifungal powder to your feet and sprinkle some in your gym shoes.
- Cover workout mats with a towel. It will protect you from dirt and germs on the mats.
- Always wash your hands before and after using the washroom.
- Baking soda is a multipurpose cleaner for gym gear: sprinkle it in gym bags and shoes to keep them smelling fresh.
- Be considerate. Don't go to the gym when you are sick.
- Remember to clean your water bottle after each training session. Bacteria and mold can build up very quickly inside dirty water bottles. Wash with hot water and dish detergent and air dry.

*****

RECREATIONAL FACILITIES

Swimming

Swimming is a great way to get exercise, relax and have fun. We don't usually associate swimming with contracting an infectious disease, but there are hazards that we need to be aware of. It is true that the risk of contracting a swimming-related infection is relatively low. This is due mainly to the use of modern disinfection systems in swimming pools, and environmental improvements in rivers, lakes and oceans over the last few decades.

Outbreaks of illness associated with swimming and other water activities still occur. These illnesses are collectively referred to as recreational water illnesses, RWIs for short. They are caused by swallowing, breathing, or having contact with germ-contaminated water from swimming pools, hot tubs, lakes, rivers, or the sea.

Common RWIs include:

- skin infections;
- ear infections;
- respiratory infections;
- eye infections;
- wound infections; and
- diarrhea.

Diarrhea is the most prevalent RWI. It can be caused by parasites such as *Cryptosporidium* and *Giardia*, bacteria like *Shigella* and *E. coli 0157:H7*, and other germs. These germs can be found in swimming pools, hot tubs, spas, the ocean, lakes, rivers, and decorative water fountains.

RWIs spread because we share the water with other people. Swimmers with diarrhea can contaminate the water with their germs. Most people have trace amounts of feces on their bottoms; sometimes people, especially small children, can lose control over their bowels in the pool. Their feces can contain millions of germs that can easily contaminate large swimming pools or entire waterparks. If disinfectant is not maintained at the appropriate levels, germs can increase to the point where they can infect large numbers of swimmers.

Chlorine is the most commonly used pool disinfectant. In properly maintained pools it will kill most germs in less than an hour. It takes longer to kill parasites such as *Cryptosporidium*, which can survive for several days in chlorine-treated water.

Lakes, rivers and the sea can be contaminated by sewage spills, animal waste, industrial pollutants and run-off water following heavy rainfall. Certain germs can survive in salt water for extended periods of time.

You need to understand all the risks and take the necessary steps to protect your family from RWIs.

Pool and Waterpark Precautions

We need to take certain precautions to stop germs from causing illness at the pool and to keep germs out of the pool.

- Avoid pools that are visibly dirty, badly maintained or crowded.
- Never swallow pool water and avoid getting water in your mouth.

- Practise good personal hygiene. Take a shower before and after swimming; wash your hands after using the toilet or changing diapers.
- Wash or sanitize your hands before eating or handling food.
- Don't swim when you have diarrhea. Your germs can spread in the water and make other people sick. Keep children with diarrhea out of the water.
- Take children on regular bathroom breaks and check diapers often.
- Change diapers in a washroom, never at the poolside. Germs can spread in and around the pool and infect other swimmers.
- Clean children thoroughly before swimming, especially between the buttocks. If soap and hot water are not available, use antibacterial wipes.
- Never swim when you have an open wound or skin infection.

Hot Tub and Spa Precautions

Disinfectants like chlorine evaporate faster in hot water, making it possible for some germs to survive. Skin infections like hot tub rash are the most common RWIs found in hot tubs and spas. Germs that cause serious diseases, including acute lung infections, can also live in hot tubs. Cases have been reported of people developing pneumonia caused by *Pseudomonas aeruginosa* bacteria contracted in hot tubs. Infected people develop tuberculosis-like symptoms, including fever, chills and coughing up of blood. The bacteria can be released from water droplets, or from the steam in hot tubs, and then inhaled into the lungs.

The CDC provides these standards for hot tub safety:

- Hot tubs should contain one to three milligrams of chlorine per litre of water and should be kept at a pH level of 7.2 to 7.8. Bacteria can multiply if chlorine levels drop and pH rises.
- It is important to check disinfectant levels even more regularly than in swimming pools. Chlorine rapidly dissipates when the water temperature rises above 29° C/84° F.
- Hot tub owners should monitor pH levels regularly and make the necessary adjustments to maintain the correct level of disinfection.
- The water should be changed on a regular basis, especially after heavy use.

Lakes, Rivers and Oceans

The water in rivers, lakes and the ocean can become contaminated with germs from sewage, animal waste, fecal accidents and germs on swimmers' bodies. Never swallow the water, and avoid swimming after rainfalls or in areas identified as unsafe by local authorities. Contact the local health department for water-testing results and closures in your area.

TRAVEL

Many people mistakingly believe that the only health risks we face when traveling are traveler's diarrhea, contracted from contaminated food or water; and inhaling the stale, recirculated air inside the aircraft. While these dangers are real, and can result in serious illness, they are by no means the only health threats we face when we travel.

To begin with, we are herded together with thousands of other people inside airport buildings; then we get to spend anywhere from a few hours to a day or more with three or four hundred other people in the confined space of an aircraft. Airports and aircraft are perfect examples of high-risk areas for germ contamination. They are high-traffic gateways where a multitude of germs are deposited at any given time and transmitted to other people. People are traveling more than ever before, and to more locations. Approximately 1.8 billion people traveled on aircraft in 2004, and the number continues to increase steadily every year. More people are traveling to developing countries where emergent infections seem to originate.

Aircraft and airports have become the transmission channels of choice for many germs. Bacteria, viruses, fungi and parasites exist to multiply and fill the earth. What better way for them to do so than to use the most modern, fastest and farthest reaching means of transportation available, not unlike what humans do. The interior of the average aircraft represents a closed environment that is ideal for disease transmission and travelers are mixing with people from a wide geographic area.

As if this weren't enough, we often end up in parts of the world where we are exposed to a whole new array of microbial enemies. Many of these pathogens may be completely harmless to the local population, because of natural resistance built up over generations, and they may not even be aware that an infection risk exists. But a virus or bacteria that is perfectly harmless to those who have developed immunity, can make you seriously ill or kill you. These germs may be present in the drinking water, food and in the environment without local people being aware of it, since they are not getting sick.

Social customs in some places can expose you to health risks; for example, eating from communal bowls or greeting others with a kiss. Hygiene and food safety standards vary from country to country, and are non-existent in some places. This puts travelers at a higher risk for contracting a foodborne illness. Certain traditional dishes, especially those made with uncooked meat, seafood or eggs, can make unsuspecting tourists very sick.

Another risk stems from the fact that some people tend to let their guard down when on vacation. They seem to pay less attention to health hazards than they

TRAVEL

would in the relative safety of their hometowns, at precisely the time when they should be extra vigilant. It is human nature to assume nothing bad will happen because you are on vacation. But this is not true. Illness or tragedy can strike anybody, anywhere, at any time.

Arriving in a strange country at the end of a long flight can be overwhelming. We are bombarded with many different sights and sounds, we worry about our luggage and getting to the hotel, and often we have to overcome a language barrier. All these distractions can make us feel disoriented, and it becomes difficult to remain alert and recognize hazardous conditions. In addition, while we recover from jet lag and adjust to the local climate, the body's natural defence against infection may be lower and we could be at a higher risk of becoming ill.

A visit to a hospital, clinic or doctor for a medical emergency can be very dangerous in some countries. We don't like to consider that we may require medical attention while on vacation. For most people planning for medical emergencies abroad begins and ends with taking out insurance coverage. Many countries have medical services and facilities that compare favourably with those in North America. Sadly, too many other countries lack the facilities and trained personnel to provide safe and efficient medical care to either local residents or tourists. In some places hospitals and clinics are downright dangerous places where infectious diseases like hepatitis and septicemia run rampant.

Cruise ships promise a relaxing, romantic and carefree vacation on the high seas. Millions of people enjoy cruises every year. Unfortunately, cruise ships also provide very favourable conditions for outbreaks of infectious diseases. Irrespective of how big a cruise ship is, it remains a confined space with a lot of people inside; in other words, a high-traffic, highly contaminated area. Traveling with lots of people in confined spaces can expose you to contaminated food, water and infectious diseases. Add the carefree holiday spirit that prevails, increased alcohol consumption and the round-the-clock buffet style of food service found on most cruise ships, and you have the perfect formula for infectious disease outbreaks. It should come as no surprise that thousands of people get sick aboard cruise ships each year from Norwalk virus and other infectious diseases.

I am not suggesting that you forfeit that once in a lifetime opportunity to go on a cruise. But I do urge caution and vigilance. It is possible to avoid infectious germs and stay healthy on board a cruise ship if you apply all the rules for basic hygiene, food safety and the safe use of public washrooms.

Cross-country train or bus journeys pose many of the same risks to your health. See the chapter on *Public Transportation* for an overview of the general precautions you can take to prevent contact with infectious germs on a bus or train. Exercise caution when eating in a train dining car, always keep your hands clean and germ-free, and use toilets with extreme caution.

When we travel to other parts of the world we could also be exposed to different strains of common infections like colds or seasonal flu. Having had the flu at home doesn't mean you are immune to all flu viruses.

When considering all the health threats and other dangers when traveling, one could be forgiven for thinking that it's best never to leave the house. For many people, to stop traveling is not an option. Life would be a lot less interesting and exciting if we stopped traveling to other countries.

Fortunately for us, common sense once again comes to the rescue. We cannot eliminate every single risk when traveling, but by understanding the dangers and by taking a number of easy, inexpensive and practical precautions, we can reduce the risk of contracting infectious disease by a wide margin.

Before You Leave

Learn as much as possible about any country you intend to visit. Pay attention to local customs, food and traditions. It is worth investing in a good travel guide-book. Talk to your travel agent and friends or relatives who have visited your planned destination. Do research on the Internet. The time spent on research can save your vacation, or your life.

Most people do a really good job researching all the tourist attractions and best places to stay, and finding the best deals on flights and accommodation. These are all valuable things to do to prepare for a vacation, but too many people fail to pay the same attention to the risk of infectious diseases at their intended destination.

Make sure you gather accurate information on the food safety risks that exist in the countries you plan to visit. Know in advance what to expect, and, more

SURVIVAL OF THE CLEANEST

importantly, what to avoid. If you are traveling to high-risk destinations, pack your own food. High energy snack foods, dried fruit, nuts and dehydrated backpacker meals are nutritious, lightweight and won't spoil. Even if you plan to eat the local food, it's a good idea to pack at least enough food for one meal a day for emergencies, or in case you get sick from the local fare. Be sure to take enough energy drink mix. Energy drinks contain sugars and sodium that work better to rehydrate the body than water.

Put together a *travel survival pack*. Include at least the following items:

- hand sanitizer gel;
- antibacterial wipes;
- heavy duty facial tissues;
- antibacterial liquid soap;
- water filter and purifier;
- disinfectant spray and/or wipes;
- basic first aid kit;
- disposable latex or plastic gloves;
- insect repellent; and
- disposable face masks.

If you are traveling to countries where medical facilities are unsafe, add these items:

- sealed, disposable hypodermic syringes and needles;
- at least one intravenous fluid kit; and
- a suture kit.

Boost your immune system before leaving. Eat a healthy diet with plenty of fruit and vegetables, take vitamin supplements and get enough sleep and exercise. These steps will not only reduce your risk of infection, but will also help you cope better with long flights and jet lag.

Place all food, water bottles, toiletries and other personal items in strong, transparent plastic bags before you pack them in your luggage. This will protect them from germs when your bags are searched.

At the Departure Airport

Don't be fooled by all the shiny glass and steel; airports are some of the most unsanitary, germ-infested places you'll ever visit. Their very reason for existence dictates that airports will be high-risk areas for infectious diseases. An airport is essentially a big and expensive funnel. Thousands of people, from many different places, pass through the funnel daily, on their way to other destinations. And, in the process, they leave behind a frightening diversity of germs on every surface they touch, sneeze or cough on, or otherwise pollute.

Any facility, object or surface in an airport should be approached with extreme caution. There are a number of common sense rules that will protect you and your family from infection in airports.

The *first* rule is to always assume that any object or surface inside an airport building has been contaminated with a variety of harmful germs. Public washrooms in airports are very scary places. They should be used with the utmost caution. Follow *all* the rules for safely using public washrooms as described in the chapter on *Public Washrooms*. Follow these rules to the letter. Public telephones, automated banking machines and vending machines should be used with extreme caution and avoided if possible. Always wash and disinfect your hands after using these facilities. Telephone handsets should be sanitized with disinfectant spray or wipes before use. Follow the contact time recommendations for the product you use.

Passports, tickets and boarding passes are handled by many different people during check-in and security procedures and become contaminated with germs as a result. Always wash and/or sanitize your hands after handling any of these items. Better still, place them inside protective clear plastic covers that can be cleaned with a disinfectant wipe.

The *second* rule is to be careful with what you eat or drink at airports. Do not eat any high-risk foods, or foods that you are not used to. Avoid chicken, seafood (cooked or raw) and dishes made with eggs or dairy products. Don't eat undercooked red meat, especially hamburger meat. Whenever possible, avoid eating at airports altogether. Eat a good meal at home before leaving for the airport, or pack your own food or snacks. Never use a drinking fountain or drink water from a tap in an airport. Take your own water or buy bottled water. When you do eat at an airport, be sure to follow the food safety guidelines described in the chapter on *Food Safety*.

Rule *three* is to be extremely diligent about keeping your hands clean. You can never be too careful at an airport.

TRAVEL

Don't go near an airport without sufficient hand sanitizer gel and antibacterial wipes. I also recommend keeping a few disposable gloves handy. Wash and sanitize your hands frequently and be very conscious to never touch your eyes, nose or mouth while you are inside an airport. Never eat without washing *and* sanitizing your hands. At a minimum, always wash and/or sanitize your hands:

- after pushing a luggage cart;
- after checking in;
- after going through security checks;
- before and after using the washroom;
- after shopping;
- after using telephones, banking or vending machines;
- after handling money or credit cards;
- after handling a passport, ticket or boarding pass;
- after touching elevator buttons or escalator rails;
- after reading a newspaper or magazine; and
- after boarding your flight.

On Board the Aircraft

There are a number of common sense rules for avoiding infectious disease on board an aircraft.

- **Be prepared** – Make sure that you have everything you will need to stay germ-free and comfortable during the flight within easy reach. I use a compact nylon bag that fits in the seatback storage pocket. It can hold a few small bottles of hand sanitizer gel,

SURVIVAL OF THE CLEANEST

antibacterial wipes, eye drops, nasal spray, ear plugs, a compact toothbrush and toothpaste, gum, lip balm, any medication I may need, plastic bandages, disinfectant wipes, my passport, tickets and a pen.

- **Take control of your immediate environment** – As we have seen in the *Basic Rules* chapter, we take control of our environment by cleaning and disinfecting any surfaces we are likely to come into contact with. The very first thing to do once you have found your seat is to disinfect your entire seating area. Use disinfectant wipes to clean and sanitize the armrests, fold-down tray, seat belt buckle, audio/video console buttons, touch screen display, air vent knob and window shutter. This will remove any germs deposited by previous passengers. Clean your hands with an antibacterial wipe and apply hand sanitizer gel when you're finished.

- **Avoid touching any areas you don't control** – Don't touch anything unless you absolutely have to. Always wear long pants, long sleeves and closed shoes when flying. Never walk around the aircraft barefoot or in your socks. Don't hesitate to wear disposable gloves to protect your hands, especially when going to the toilet. Never lie down in the aisle to sleep. Don't sit or kneel on the floor. Take your own pillow, headphones or headphone covers. Never use the heated moist towels distributed on some flights; only use the moist towels that come sealed in individual plastic pouches. Better yet, use your own antibacterial wipes.

TRAVEL

- **Keep your hands clean and germ-free at all times** – This is the single most important step you can take to avoid getting sick during a flight. Always clean and disinfect your hands on board an aircraft:
  - before and after eating;
  - after reading the in-flight magazine; and
  - before and after using the washroom.

- **Eating and drinking** – Do not assume that food and water aboard commercial aircraft are safe. Food and water are obtained in the country of departure where different food safety standards apply and may be contaminated. NEVER drink the water that comes from aircraft tanks. The water is not safe!

  During November and December of 2004, the US Environmental Protection Agency (EPA) conducted a water quality sampling of 169 aircraft at 12 airports. They took water samples from galley water taps and lavatory faucets from each aircraft. The EPA found that the water on 17.2% of these aircraft (29 aircraft) tested positive for coliform bacteria. Coliforms are a group of related bacteria found in the environment and in the digestive tracts of humans and other warm-blooded animals. While the presence of coliforms is not necessarily a health risk, the presence of coliform bacteria in drinking water means that other infectious germs may be present.

  Request bottled or canned beverages while on the aircraft and refrain from drinking tea or coffee not made with bottled water. The water used to prepare coffee and tea aboard an airplane is generally not brought to

SURVIVAL OF THE CLEANEST

a sufficiently high temperature to guarantee that all germs are killed. I strongly advise against eating airline food, and not just because it typically tastes awful. The mass, industrial-style production and distribution of airline food, the way it is stored and handled on board aircraft, and the cramped, unsanitary conditions in the passenger area where meals are served all invite contamination.

Eat before taking off on a short flight; pack your own food for longer flights. If eating airline food cannot be avoided, because of very long flights or for other reasons, several precautions are required to avoid getting sick:

- Avoid high-risk foods like chicken, fish or dairy.
- Disinfect your hands after opening the packaging on the food tray and before eating.
- If the food doesn't smell or look right, don't eat it.

■ **Aircraft toilets** – Public toilets are dangerous places at the best of times; aircraft interiors are unsanitary germ traps. It follows that aircraft toilets are the most unhealthy, germ-infested places in the universe. Several factors combine to contaminate aircraft toilets: high traffic, confined space, mix of people, varied levels of hygiene among passengers, lack of consideration for others, and inadequate cleaning and sanitizing. There are no redeeming factors I can think of. Always follow the golden rules described below:

- *First golden rule* for aircraft toilets: Never, *never* touch anything with your bare hands or any part of your body. Never. Push the door open with your shoe, or cover your hand with a disposable glove, paper towel, napkin or heavy duty facial tissue before touching the door. Once inside, keep your hands covered when you lock the door, and when you operate faucets and soap dispensers. Do not sit down directly on the toilet seat – EVER! Follow *all* the steps for using public toilets as described in *Public Washrooms*. Don't touch anything directly on your way out.

- *Second golden rule*: Always wash *and* sanitize your hands when using an aircraft toilet. Do not rely on hand washing only on board an aircraft; the water may be contaminated with germs. Wash your hands *and* sanitize with sanitizing gel or wipes before touching your genitals or any part of your body. Wash *and* sanitize your hands after using the toilet. Be very careful to avoid recontaminating your hands. Always take the precautions described in *Basic Rules*. Sanitize your hands again when you have returned to your seat. *You can never be too careful when using an aircraft toilet!*

- *Third golden rule*: Never drink water from the faucet in an aircraft toilet, or use it to brush your teeth or wash your face. In addition to the high levels of germs present in aircraft tank water, washroom faucets are some of the most contaminated surfaces in the entire aircraft. Use bottled water to brush your teeth and use pre-moistened disposable cloths to clean your face.

■ **Protect your eyes, nose and mouth** – The eyes, nose and mouth are weak links in the body's anti-germ armour. Most infectious diseases begin when germs enter the body via one or more of these portals. We need to take extra precautions to protect these areas from germs; more so when we find ourselves in a high-risk environment like an aircraft cabin. Avoid touching your eyes, nose or mouth. This action transfers germs from your hands, to parts of the body more vulnerable to infection. Many people are not aware that they touch their eyes, noses or mouths; it requires a conscious effort to stop doing so. Ask a friend or relative to tell you when you touch your face. Once you are aware of your actions they become easier to control. If you habitually rub or pick at your eyes, wear glasses when you travel, even if you don't need corrective lenses. Wear a disposable face mask if you can't avoid touching your nose or mouth. A face mask also provides some protection against airborne germs.

- **Don't dehydrate** – Moist membranes inside the nasal passages provide protection against germs. These membranes can dry out rapidly in the drying air inside an aircraft. Dry membranes become cracked and open to infection. The best defence is to keep well hydrated and to use a moisturizing spray in your nose. Nasal sprays have the added advantage of flushing away germs. In addition to being uncomfortable and irritating, dry eyes may also be more vulnerable to infection. Use lubricating eye drops when you fly. You're also more likely to rub and touch dry, irritated eyes. Always clean and disinfect your hands before administering eye drops or nasal spray.

- **Protect any areas of broken skin** – Never leave any cuts, nicks, burns or other areas of broken skin unprotected. Ensure that any existing injuries are treated and covered before you board, and that they remain covered throughout the flight. If you cut, scratch or otherwise injure yourself during the flight, clean and protect the area immediately. Rinse the wound with bottled water or an alcoholic beverage. Never rinse it under the tap in the aircraft toilet. Disinfect the area with an antibacterial wipe or sanitizing gel, or use a wound disinfectant if available. Cover with a plastic bandage. I prefer the brands that have an antibacterial agent applied to the wound pad. They provide added protection against infection. Leaving damaged skin unprotected in an aircraft can be a deadly mistake.

- **Report unsanitary conditions** – Don't ignore unhygienic or hazardous conditions inside the cabin. Report any problems to the cabin crew and inform other passengers as appropriate. Follow up to ensure that the issue has been resolved.

A note on fellow passengers: We cannot control how other passengers behave. Given the close proximity of the next seat, you may well be exposed to infectious germs because of other people's ignorance and lack of consideration. There are a number of things you can do to mitigate your risk of infection by association.

Do not hesitate to share your knowledge of preventive hygiene. Quite often, people act in a certain way because they are unaware of the health risks. By setting an example, and with the right amount of tact, I have converted a fair number of fellow passengers to the 'Survival' approach. Don't be obnoxious or a bore. One approach that I found works really well is to offer sanitizer gel or an antibacterial wipe at an appropriate time, such as when meals or drinks are served. This usually breaks the ice and provides an opening to start talking about the dangers of germs and infectious disease aboard commercial aircraft. I always pack extra hand sanitizer gel and wipes to give away to people seated next to me. This not only makes their flight safer, but it also helps to break the chain of infection on board the aircraft.

On the other hand, if the person in the next seat does something really unhygienic, inconsiderate or gross, do not hesitate to speak up, even if it means being rude. If he or she refuses to cooperate, involve the cabin crew. Nobody has the right to expose you to infectious disease through their behaviour.

At Destination or Connecting Airports

Do *not* let down your guard when you arrive at your destination airport or at a connecting airport. Practise the same diligence and take the precautions described in the *departure airport* section above. Approach washrooms with caution, be careful where and what you eat, and avoid handling or touching anything with your bare hands.

At Your Vacation Destination

After leaving the airport, your first exposure to infectious disease will most likely come from whatever form of public transportation you use to get to your hotel or resort. The chapter on *Public Transportation* provides detailed steps for safely using public buses, subways, trains and taxis. Follow these guidelines carefully. Always practise common sense and follow the basic rules of preventive hygiene.

When you get to your hotel, guesthouse, resort or other accommodation, you are still at risk from germs. Never assume that everything is clean and germ-free. Before you unpack, use the bathroom, eat, drink or do anything else, always disinfect all high-risk surfaces and objects. Use disinfectant spray or wipes (you *did* remember to pack some?) to sanitize the toilet seat, flushing handle, sink, countertops, faucets, the bathtub or shower cubicle, and bathroom doorhandle. Disinfect any tabletops, counters and shelves where you are likely to eat or store food, cosmetics or toiletries. Wash any glasses, cups or eating utensils provided in the room with hot water. Run taps for at least two minutes to get rid of dirt and germs that may have colonized the inside of the plumbing. If the tap water is suspect, boil water to disinfect the utensils, or use a solution with water purification tablets or drops. You can also use antibacterial hand soap to wash dishes, just remember to rinse well. Check that the linen and towels are clean and fresh; if not, don't hesitate to ask for replacements.

Never go anywhere without sufficient hand sanitizer gel, antibacterial wipes, and disinfectant spray or wipes. It is a common custom in many countries to greet other people, including strangers, with a handshake. Quite often this cannot be avoided without offending the other person. Always clean and sanitize your hands as soon as possible after shaking hands; apply sanitizer gel if you are not able to wash your hands. Your hands are microbial minefields. They should always be treated as contaminated and dangerous. When in doubt, wash and sanitize.

Food and Drink

Food safety rules continue to apply when you're on vacation. The rules don't change just because you are on vacation; the dangers of foodborne disease do not disappear either. If anything, you need to be more vigilant and careful. Always exercise extreme caution with food and drink when traveling. Eating contaminated food can do more than just spoil your vacation: it can cause illness that can permanently damage your health, or even cost you your life.

Contaminated food and drink are common sources for the introduction of infection into the body. Among the more common infectious diseases that travelers can acquire from contaminated food and drink are *E. coli* infections, shigellosis or bacillary dysentery, giardiasis, cryptosporidiosis, Norwalk virus, and hepatitis A. Other infectious disease risks for travelers include typhoid fever and other salmonellosis, cholera, and rotavirus infections. Many of the infectious diseases transmitted in food and water can also be acquired directly through contact with fecal matter.

Virtually all foods and beverages are subject to contamination. The risk increases with raw or undercooked foods. Avoid raw and undercooked meat, fish, shellfish and other seafood, salads and uncooked vegetables, unpasteurized milk and other dairy products such as cream. Stick to food that has been properly cooked and is still piping hot, or fruit and vegetables that you have washed and peeled personally. In places where hygiene and sanitation are suspect, high-risk foods like chicken, seafood and dairy products should be avoided entirely.

Cooked food that has been left out at ambient temperatures provides a fertile environment for bacteria. Don't go near it!

DO NOT buy food and beverages from street food vendors when traveling in developing countries. Street vendor food probably makes more tourists ill in any given year than all other travel-related causes combined. You should never buy high-risk food from any street vendor, even in countries with strict food safety standards.

Chlorinating water at the correct levels, and following water treatment practices similar to those used in Canada and the United States, will provide substantial protection against most viral and bacterial waterborne diseases. However, chlorine treatment on its own, as used in the disinfection of municipal water, might not kill some enteric viruses and the parasitic organisms that cause giardiasis and cryptosporidiosis. In areas where chlorinated tap water is not available or where hygiene and sanitation are poor, only the following might be safe to drink:

- Hot beverages, such as tea and coffee, made with boiled water or bottled water.

SURVIVAL OF THE CLEANEST

- Canned or bottled carbonated beverages, including carbonated bottled water and soft drinks.
- Beer and wine.

Street vendors in some countries refill used soft drink bottles with their own concoctions and sell them to unsuspecting tourists. Bottled water offered by some vendors is often unsafe tap water in non-sterile, used plastic bottles. Make sure you carry plenty of clean, safe drinking water with you so that you're not tempted to buy water or other beverages on the street. Buy water, pop or juice at a grocery store or at your hotel before heading out. Always check all bottled beverages to ensure that cap seals are intact.

Where water might be contaminated, ice should also be considered contaminated and should not be used in beverages. If ice has been in contact with containers used for drinking, thoroughly clean the containers, preferably with soap and hot water. Your safest bet is avoiding ice altogether when traveling.

It is safer to drink a beverage directly from the can or bottle than from a questionable drinking glass. However, water on the outside of beverage cans or bottles may also be contaminated. Always dry wet cans or bottles before they are opened and wipe clean surfaces with which the mouth will have direct contact. Better still, use an alcohol wipe for extra insurance. Never brush your teeth with tap water that is not safe to drink.

Water can be treated to make it safe for drinking and other uses by boiling, filtration, or chemical purification. Please see the chapter on *Drinking Water* for details.

TRAVEL

When traveling to more challenging countries, I pack my own cutlery, plastic cup and glass. Utensils from picnic or camping sets work well; they're compact, lightweight and will withstand the rigours of travel. Whenever you are not comfortable using the utensils in a restaurant, use your own. Don't worry if other people think your behaviour a bit strange; they'll get over it.

Never eat from a communal bowl or plate, and don't drink from shared cups, bottles or any other container. No matter how exotic or romantic such settings may appear in travel programs or movies; it is not worth the risk to your health. One handful of food can contain sufficient germs to bring down a small army with diseases like dysentery, hepatitis, cholera, typhoid or other equally deadly infections. Avoid places and situations where shared meals are served. If you do find yourself in a situation where it is impossible to avoid sharing in a communal meal, or if it is the only food that stands between you and starvation, proceed with extreme caution. Try to take food from a part of the bowl that hasn't been touched by anybody else and avoid high-risk dishes like chicken and seafood. Stick to the foods least popular with the other diners.

There is no safe way to drink from a shared cup, jug, bottle or bowl. If you can't avoid accepting an offered drink without offending your host, put up a good show of pretending to drink without actually doing so, or touching your lips against the rim of the container.

When you buy fruit and vegetables, particularly from street vendors or markets, ensure that you wash them properly before eating. Only use water that is safe enough to drink for washing produce. If clean water is unavailable, an antibacterial wipe can be used to clean fruit or vegetables. Peeling produce will also remove contaminants. Remember to wash the produce first; peeling can transfer surface germs to the rest of the fruit. The most effective way to clean and sanitize produce is to soak and wash it in a water purifier and filtered water solution. Soak for 20 minutes, wash, rinse with clean solution and air dry. I use this method when traveling.

Taking all these precautions may seem like a lot of work. Rest assured, it's not. They quickly become second nature and part of your normal travel routine. Don't forget, getting sick always takes more time out of your life. Very few people have unlimited vacation time; don't let illness spoil your hard-earned holiday. Encourage your family or travel partners to acquire the same safe travel habits. One person's illness can spoil the trip for everybody.

Traveler's Diarrhea

Traveler's diarrhea is the collective term for the illness caused by bacteria, protozoa, or viruses ingested by consuming food or water that has been contaminated by fecal matter. Two types of traveler's diarrhea, cholera and giardiasis, can be fatal.

People who travel to countries with poor public sanitation and hygiene are most at risk. With some exceptions, developing countries located in Africa, Asia, and Latin America are high-risk areas for contracting traveler's diarrhea. Symptoms include nausea, severe

TRAVEL

cramps, bloating, watery stools, fatigue and headache. Dehydration can also be a serious and fatal side effect.

Most cases of traveler's diarrhea can be prevented by taking a few basic precautions.

- Don't drink the tap water! Use bottled water, boil or chemically treat water for:
  - drinking, mixing drinks or making coffee and tea;
  - brushing your teeth;
  - washing your face and hands;
  - washing fruit and vegetables;
  - washing eating and cooking utensils; and
  - cleaning food and beverage containers.
- Avoid raw food. Any uncooked food could be contaminated, including:
  - fruit, vegetables and salad greens;
  - unpasteurized milk and milk products;
  - meat, poultry, fish and shellfish.
- Do not buy food from street vendors.
- Avoid food buffets.
- Don't eat any moist food at room temperature.
- Eat only fruit and vegetables that you have peeled yourself. Avoid salads and fruit that cannot be peeled.
- Drink canned or bottled drinks from the container, after wiping it clean and only if you have broken the seal yourself.
- Avoid ice cubes and fresh fruit juices.

SURVIVAL OF THE CLEANEST

- Tea, coffee and other hot beverages ordered in a restaurant should be steaming hot.
- Keep your mouth closed in the shower.
- Do not swim in lakes or rivers that may be contaminated with fecal matter.
- Wash and sanitize your hands! Never eat or handle food with dirty hands.

If you do get sick, remember to drink plenty of non-contaminated fluids to prevent dehydration. Seek medical attention if your diarrhea is severe or if it continues for more than three days.

Shopping

Take care when buying curios, craft, art and other items from street markets or vendors. These items are handled by many browsing tourists, and they are not always made or stored in the most sanitary conditions. Some craft items are made with animal or plant components that could be contaminated or even poisonous. Be sure to clean and disinfect your hands after handling any items while shopping or browsing. When you return to your lodging, clean and disinfect any items that won't be damaged by the process or cleaning products; seal other objects in plastic bags and avoid handling them as far as possible. Disinfectant sprays are useful for sanitizing items with irregular surfaces or hard-to-reach areas. Be sure to check that the active ingredients in the disinfectant won't harm your purchase. Read the label and always test on a small, hidden area.

Injuries, Cuts, Burns and Rashes

Treat and cover any areas of broken skin immediately. Always carry a basic first aid kit that includes an antiseptic lotion and plastic bandages. Follow the steps described in *Basic Rules*.

A note on sexually transmitted diseases:

It is outside the scope of this book to discuss sexually transmitted diseases or other medical issues, and it is most definitely not my intention to make any kind of moral judgment or statement. However, reality and common sense dictate that extreme caution should be used regarding sexual contact when traveling. It becomes more critical when traveling to parts of the world where HIV/AIDS, hepatitis and other sexually transmitted diseases are prevalent. Consider the risks and consequences carefully before you decide to engage in sexual contact with strangers. If you decide to engage in casual sex during your vacation, exercise the utmost caution and do everything possible to protect yourself, not only from sexual diseases, but also from the other infectious diseases associated with close contact with other people.

Animals

Avoid contact with domestic and wild animals while traveling. Animals carry a wide range of harmful germs, including the deadly rabies virus. In addition to rabies, bites and scratches from dogs, cats and other animals can cause infections and serious diseases like tetanus.

SURVIVAL OF THE CLEANEST

Avoid touching pets, farm animals and animals in petting zoos. Bacteria like *E. coli* thrive on animals. Always wash or sanitize your hands thoroughly after touching or handling any animals. The same applies when riding on horses, donkeys, camels, elephants, llamas, ostriches, etc. Wear long pants and sleeves, don't touch your face, wash and disinfect your hands and shower and change your clothes as soon as possible.

For more information on animal-borne infections please see *Pets & Wild Animals*.

Medical Emergencies

If you or a family member require medical attention while traveling, always exercise the utmost caution and stick to the guidelines in the *Medical Facilities* chapter. Do not seek medical help for every minor illness or injury; unnecessary visits to hospitals or doctors increase your risk for more serious infections. If you are traveling to developing countries that lack proper medical facilities (many do, unfortunately), pack some basic medical supplies. At a minimum, include a few sealed, sterile hypodermic syringes; one or more intravenous fluid kits; a suture kit; bandages; and lots of disinfectant. If there is a high likelihood of getting into an accident or suffering a serious injury during your travels, consider taking a blood plasma kit to avoid the risks associated with blood transfusions in some countries. Learn how to use these things correctly! Consult your doctor about getting a prescription for a broad spectrum antibiotic to use in an emergency. Ask your doctor for a letter to confirm that the medical supplies in your possession are for legitimate reasons, otherwise you may have problems when clearing customs.

If you are taking any prescription drugs, make sure you have enough for the duration of your trip and a few extra days.

Cruise Ships

More than eight million cruise ship passengers embark from North American ports every year. Worldwide, ten million passengers travel on cruise ships annually. Large cruise ships crowd thousands of passengers into confined areas, where interaction with other people is impossible to avoid. Passengers take part in on-board activities, and food is served in communal areas. Passengers and crew members on cruise ships come from all over the globe; their personal hygiene norms, immunization status, behaviour and their potential as disease carriers vary widely. Cruise ships move rapidly from one port to another, exposing passengers and crew to different sanitation standards and infectious disease risks. Diseases can spread quickly to other passengers and crew members on board the ship. Disembarking passengers and crew members can spread these diseases in their communities when they return home.

Any infectious disease can easily spread on board a cruise ship. The list of reported outbreaks include: measles, rubella, varicella, meningococcal meningitis, hepatitis A, Legionnaire's disease, and a variety of respiratory and gastrointestinal illnesses. Influenza and

SURVIVAL OF THE CLEANEST

Norwalk virus outbreaks have occurred frequently in the last couple of years.

You can protect your health by taking a few precautions:

- Ensure that all your routine vaccinations are up to date. Follow the vaccination recommendations that apply to each country on your cruise.
- Wash your hands frequently: before and after eating, before and after using the toilet, after using any shared facilities, after touching high-traffic surfaces such as guardrails and doorhandles, after shaking somebody's hand, and whenever your hands are sticky or dirty.
- Use an alcohol-based hand sanitizer in addition to regular hand washing and don't touch your face.
- Follow all the precautions in the *Food Safety* chapter. Approach food buffets with extreme caution. Avoid high-risk foods such as raw shellfish, chicken, and undercooked meat and seafood dishes.
- Stick to the rules for using *Public Washrooms*.
- Avoid people who sneeze or cough. Immediately leave the area if someone throws up. Be sure to inform a crew member.
- Drink plenty of water. Drinking water prevents dehydration and keeps mucous membranes moist. Dry membranes become cracked and susceptible to infection.
- Be considerate towards others. If you become ill before a cruise, cancel your trip or reschedule. If you get sick on board, stay in your cabin.

CAMPING & OUTDOORS

Ironically, primitive wilderness camping is safer from an infectious disease perspective than 'civilized' camping in fully serviced campgrounds. This is true for two reasons: first, people are the most important vectors in the spread of harmful germs; the farther we get away from close contact with other people, the lower our risk of infection. Secondly, we don't share washrooms and other facilities with fellow campers when we camp in unserviced wilderness areas.

Does this mean we can abandon personal hygiene and stop being concerned about infectious disease when we camp in the backcountry? Of course not! Germs are everywhere, and many bacteria, viruses, fungi and parasites that occur in the natural environment will thrive in unclean conditions and pose a threat to our health. Failing to keep hands clean and handle food safely have made many a camper seriously ill. Minor cuts and scrapes can become infected wounds if left untreated. Paying attention to the safety of drinking water becomes more important in the wilderness.

A relatively minor illness or infection can become life-threatening if you are far away from medical assistance. Infections can weaken you, limit your mobility and affect your ability to think clearly in emergency situations. Besides, being sick while on a wilderness trip isn't anybody's idea of fun.

A strange thing seems to happen to some people when they are out in the wilderness. They abandon basic hygiene and food safety practices. For some inexplicable reason they seem to think that the basic, common sense rules don't apply once they're out of the city. Big mistake! There is a very real risk of becoming infected with germs from the environment, food, water, cooking utensils and fellow campers if we don't pay attention to cleanliness in the campsite or on the trail.

For ease of reference we'll distinguish between 'civilized' camping and wilderness camping. Civilized camping is defined as camping in serviced campground facilities, typically sharing the campground and facilities with other campers. Campers have access to washrooms, kitchen facilities and sometimes laundromats and other amenities. Wilderness camping is defined as camping in the backcountry, in randomly selected sites, or in defined but unserviced campsites. These sites typically have no facilities or, at best, a pit toilet.

Civilized (Serviced) Camping

Camping in fully serviced campgrounds is a popular way of vacationing for many North American families. It offers families most of the comforts of other forms of holiday accommodation without the expense of hotels or condo rentals, or the inconvenience and high fuel costs of towing a trailer or driving an RV.

CAMPING & OUTDOORS

Serviced campgrounds typically provide washrooms with showers, and many have shared kitchen facilities. Some also have laundromats, convenience stores, TV and games rooms, and swimming pools or hot tubs. They enable us to get away and still have all the creature comforts, or most of them at least.

Serviced campgrounds provide individuals and families alike with fun and affordable holidays. Having said that, we cannot, and should not, ignore the fact that campground facilities can harbour infectious disease and make campers and their families seriously ill. Like all shared facilities, surface areas can become contaminated with other people's germs very quickly and infect unsuspecting campers. And, as is the case with all public facilities, levels of cleanliness, the standards of hygiene and the quality of service can vary greatly from one campground to the next.

Problems with cleanliness and germ contamination increase dramatically during the busy summer holidays when campgrounds are packed and service staff battle to keep up with cleaning and maintenance chores.

With many people using communal facilities in a campground, it is unrealistic to assume that everybody will have the same high standards of cleanliness that you do, or that your fellow campers are even aware of the health risks they face or cause through their ignorant behaviour. We have to take responsibility for preventing infection when camping and for protecting our families' health and safety.

Having read a number of the other chapters in the book, you are well aware by now that the theme of the book is not to avoid public places or enjoyable activities like camping, but rather to provide a balanced and common sense approach to preventing infection. It follows that I am not advocating shutting down all public campgrounds or that we never go camping again. By using good old common sense, and by taking a few simple precautions, you and your family can enjoy a relaxed camping holiday and take advantage of the facilities provided at serviced campgrounds.

The following guidelines provide the road map for safe and enjoyable camping:

- **Be selective** – Choose campgrounds with a reputation for neatness, cleanliness and good service.
- **Do your homework** – Research several campgrounds in the area where you are planning to vacation. Ask for and check references, talk to friends, colleagues or relatives who are familiar with the campgrounds you consider visiting, and check with local authorities for any campground health and safety violations on their records. If you are planning to camp close to home, visit the campground prior to making your reservation. Do not be afraid to ask direct questions when talking to campground managers. Ask about washroom cleaning schedules, garbage facilities, pool maintenance schedules, and general maintenance and cleaning services. Choose another campground if your questions are not answered to your satisfaction. Vague or dismissive responses are good indicators of problems and a lack of good facilities management.

CAMPING & OUTDOORS

- **Inspect first** – Upon arrival, do a quick visual inspection of the campground before paying your fee or setting up camp. Take a few minutes to inspect the washrooms, kitchen and other common areas. It's usually a bad sign if your request for an inspection is denied; go somewhere else. Things to be on the lookout for include overflowing trash cans, dirty or foul-smelling washrooms, litter lying around the campground, greasy or dirty countertops in the kitchen area, and dirt, litter or bad smells in communal recreation areas.
- **Pick a good spot** – Once you have confirmed that the campground meets your high standards for cleanliness, the next step is to pick a good place to set up camp. Select a site that is as far away as possible from the washrooms, kitchen and any other common areas. Also avoid sites that are on or near heavily traveled paths, such as those to and from shared facilities or the parking lot. That way you will avoid the smells and litter associated with washrooms, kitchens and other shared areas. As an added bonus, you'll also enjoy more peace, quiet and privacy. Also avoid sites near garbage disposal bins.
- **Inspect your campsite** – Before pitching the tent and setting up your camp, carefully inspect the area for any litter, particularly food packaging, dog waste or hazardous objects like broken glass and tin cans. Sadly, finding used needles and condoms in what were traditionally family campgrounds is part of today's reality, so be careful. Safely remove and

SURVIVAL OF THE CLEANEST

dispose of any dangerous objects and keep small children away until the area is cleaned up.

- **Keep your campsite clean** – A clean, tidy and well-organized campsite is a lot easier to keep germ-free. As a bonus, there will be less clutter to trip over and things will be easier to find.
- **Stay clean** – Practise good personal hygiene around the camp. Wash your hands often and thoroughly; ensure that other members of the group, especially small children, do the same. Keep sufficient disinfectant wipes and hand sanitizer gel within easy reach around the campsite. Shower and change your clothes frequently. In addition to keeping your body germ-free, it will also be a lot more pleasant for your fellow campers to be near you. The same goes for brushing your teeth and flossing: just because you are on vacation doesn't mean dental hygiene is no longer important. Besides, your fellow campers will appreciate your fresh breath!
- **Food safety** – Always handle and store food safely. This becomes more critical when camping. Food is more exposed to the environment in a typical campsite and facilities for storing and preparing food are limited compared to the average home kitchen. There is an increased risk of germs deposited on food by insects, rodents and other scavengers. Too many people throw caution and common sense to the wind when camping or on vacation, at the very time when they should be even more cautious than at home.

CAMPING & OUTDOORS

Always take these precautions when you prepare or handle food at your campsite:

- Store perishable food in a refrigerator (if available) or in a cooler box. Top up the ice or replace ice bricks frequently to ensure that cold temperatures are maintained inside the cooler.

- Clean and disinfect all areas where food is prepared or consumed. A plastic spray bottle filled with a solution of one tablespoon chlorine bleach per litre of water makes sanitizing a quick and easy task. Spray on clean surfaces and allow to dry.

- Wash and disinfect dishes properly. Never go camping without at least a gallon jug of chlorine (household) bleach. It is your best ally against foodborne illness. *Always* disinfect dishes after washing when camping, no matter how clean they look. This goes for all utensils used to prepare, store or serve food. Please see the chapter on *Food Safety* for information on disinfecting dishes with bleach.

- Don't leave food out. Summer heat and direct sunlight can very quickly spoil food, even well-cooked food. In addition to heat, dust, insects and rodents can contaminate food with dirt and germs. Store cooked food and leftovers in a cooler or discard leftovers in the proper garbage disposal bin.

- Store non-perishable food properly. Use a sealable tote or heavy duty plastic bags to protect all food, spices, condiments, beverages, etc., that don't require refrigeration against airborne dirt, germs and other contaminants. Place totes or bags inside your tent or vehicle to avoid attracting animals or birds.

SURVIVAL OF THE CLEANEST

- Place a water container with an easy-to-operate spout, liquid antibacterial soap and a roll of paper towels on or near the camp table. You have to make it easy and convenient for people to wash their hands, otherwise they won't. If you prefer not to use antibacterial soap, use a regular liquid soap – not bar soap. Supervise children to ensure they keep their hands clean. Kids can spread a lot of germs around very quickly.
- Do not allow any person in your group to eat or handle food without washing his or her hands first.

■ **Keep your tent closed** – Keep the tent door or insect screen closed at all times. This will keep out debris, insects, birds, rodents and other animals. If it is windy or dusty around your campsite, close the full tent door, not just the insect screen, and all window flaps. It's also a good idea to spray insect repellent on door and window insect screens if you are in an area with lots of mosquitoes, flies or other flying insects. Note that repellents with high DEET concentrations can damage synthetic fabrics, so test it on a small hidden area of the tent first.

■ **Keep tents and other camping gear clean and free of mold** – Clean camping equipment after each trip and ensure that tents, fly sheets and sleeping bags are dry before storing them.

Using Shared Facilities

■ *Kitchen facilities* – I start this section with shared kitchen facilities, because what I mainly want to say about them is short and simple: Don't use them. Ever.

CAMPING & OUTDOORS

Only use them if you want to spend half your vacation cleaning and disinfecting countertops, sinks and other kitchen areas left messy and germ-ridden by other campers. Or if you want to gamble with your own or your family's health and run the risk of contracting serious foodborne or other infectious illnesses. It is easy and inexpensive to provide rudimentary kitchen facilities at your campsite for the exclusive use of your family or group. That way you avoid sharing other people's germs or becoming a victim of their bad hygiene habits.

The basic camp kitchen requires no more than a table; two or three plastic tubs for washing, rinsing and disinfecting dishes; a fuel or propane camp stove; and a couple of cooler boxes. The safest way to wash dishes in camp is to place three plastic tubs on the camp table: the first filled with plenty of hot water and a good dish soap, the second filled with clean, hot water, and the third filled with hot or cold water containing bleach (one tablespoon bleach for every gallon/3.8 litres of water). Scrape food waste into a waste container; wash the dishes in the hot, soapy water; rinse in the clean, hot water; and soak in the bleach solution for at least five minutes. Air dry the dishes on the tabletop. Never use a dishtowel. The soapy hot water will clean the dishes of dirt and food residue and the bleach solution will sanitize them by killing any germs left on the surface after washing and rinsing. It goes without saying that the tabletop should have been wiped off and sanitized before the clean dishes and utensils are laid out on the table to dry. In warm weather, with flies and other insects around, cover dishes and utensils with a suitable cloth or netting.

There really is no good reason for using shared kitchen facilities at a campground. Besides, who wants to carry food and kitchen stuff back and forth between the tent and the communal kitchen, or prepare a meal with a bunch of strange people getting in the way? If you do choose to make use of shared kitchen facilities and, again, I urge you not to, always take the following precautions:

- Avoid the rush hour. It is a matter of simple mathematics: the fewer people you share the facilities with at any given time, the lower your risk of coming into contact with infectious germs.
- Don't spare the bleach! Make sure you have enough bleach to last you for the duration of your camping vacation. Use a bleach solution of one tablespoon bleach per litre of water in a plastic spray bottle to disinfect surfaces before preparing food. Clean the surface first with a suitable cleaner and dry it thoroughly with a paper towel. Spray bleach solution on the clean surface and allow it to dry. It is your best guarantee for killing all the germs in the area. This applies to countertops, sinks, faucets, doorhandles and any surfaces that can come into contact with your food, food containers or hands. Do not even open a can of beans before you have cleaned and disinfected the entire food preparation area.
- Use only paper towels. It's not a good idea to use re-usable cloth towels to clean or wipe surfaces in a communal kitchen, or to dry your hands.

CAMPING & OUTDOORS

- Using a communal refrigerator is another big no-no. Before you can say 'E. coli,' somebody's badly packaged, week-old hamburger meat is going to leak its putrid juices straight into your freshly prepared and, up to that point, perfectly germ-free fruit salad. The closest I ever get to shared refrigeration is to use provided freezer space to store ice and to re-freeze ice bricks for my coolers. Even then, I always rinse and disinfect the ice bags and bricks before placing them in a cooler box. If you have no choice but to share a fridge with other people, double-bag your food in heavy-duty, sealable plastic bags and place it on the highest shelf, if possible. When retrieving your food, remove and discard the outer plastic bag immediately, and wash or disinfect your hands before handling the food.

- If you still insist, or feel strongly about using communal kitchen facilities, or if you find yourself in a situation where you have no choice, please familiarize yourself with the sections on safe food handling and kitchen hygiene in the *Food Safety* chapter. Follow all the guidelines meticulously, and then some!

- Do not hesitate to report any unhygienic or unsafe conditions in the kitchen area to the campground management.

■ *Washroom and shower facilities* – The washrooms at campsites are no different from any other public washrooms: The same health threats are present and the same common sense precautions apply. Please refer to *Public Washrooms* for advice on safely using public washrooms. Take extra precautions when using communal showers. Never go barefoot; wear shower shoes to protect your feet from fungal infections. Dry your feet properly after showering and apply antifungal powder for added protection. Always shower in the hottest water you can comfortably stand, and dry your body thoroughly before getting dressed. I strongly advise using a good liquid antibacterial soap.

Wilderness Camping

For many people, wilderness camping is synonymous with getting really dirty. They take it as a given that personal hygiene is going to take a backseat for a few days when they go camping or hiking in the backcountry. While it follows logically that it is more difficult to stay clean in an environment with no running water or bathroom facilities, it is by no means impossible to maintain a minimum level of cleanliness and personal hygiene, irrespective of how wild or primitive your surroundings are.

Hygiene in the wilderness is not about looking neat and clean. It is about taking basic precautions to stay healthy and comfortable, and to reduce the spread of infectious germs among people in your group. Your actions affect your own health as well as that of the friends or family with whom you are sharing the wilderness experience. Preventing infection also becomes more important if you are many miles away from the nearest town or roads, and in areas without cellular phone coverage or ranger patrols. An illness that can be readily treated under normal circumstances, can turn deadly when you are unable to get medical assistance in time. Dehydration caused by relatively harmless diarrhea can leave you too weak to hike out and seek help.

Fortunately for us, there are many innovative products available on the market today that make it really easy to stay clean and germ-free anywhere in the wilderness, even when no water is available for washing. This also means that there is no excuse for neglecting hygiene and risking your health when camping. The section below lists the basic precautions that I have found useful for avoiding harmful germs in the backwoods. As always, use common sense and be creative to adapt to the specific environment and threats you are faced with.

- **Stay as clean as possible** – Staying clean is an important part of staying healthy in the wilderness. Good personal hygiene protects you from sickness and infection, and it will make you far more popular with other people in your group! Bathe, swim or wash whenever you have the opportunity. This will remove the sweat, grime and germs that naturally build up on the body. It will also allow you the opportunity to examine yourself for signs of injury, rash, sores or ticks. You'll also feel a lot more comfortable and enjoy the trip more. Use biodegradable soap when washing or bathing in rivers or lakes to limit your impact on the environment. Specially formulated biodegradable soaps are available for washing in the ocean.

SURVIVAL OF THE CLEANEST

If water is plentiful, consider packing a camping shower. Typical models heat around four gallons of water by solar power. This is sufficient for three or four showers. The hot water can also be used for washing dishes. There are lightweight products available that fold up small enough to stow in a backpack. You'll only need one for your group, so you can take turns carrying it. To use, simply fill it with clean water and hang against a tree, tent or in any other suitable spot where it will get the maximum exposure to sunlight.

Clean up with moist antibacterial wipes or alcohol wipes if washing with water and soap is not possible. Wipes are lightweight, compact and easy to pack out with other garbage. You can remove a lot of grime from your body with one or two of these moist wipes. This will reduce chafing, body odours, and bacteria, and you will feel better if you're not sticky and grimy all over. Concentrate on keeping your hands, face, groin, feet, armpits and the areas between the buttocks clean to stay comfortable and germ-free. An inexpensive alternative is to carry a small bottle of isopropyl alcohol and some cotton pads. Soak the cotton with the alcohol and wipe your feet, groin area, between the buttocks and under your arms. The alcohol also makes a great disinfectant for treating cuts, scratches and insect bites.

- **Keep your hands clean and germ-free** – Frequent hand cleaning will prevent illness. Use water and soap if enough water is available, preferably heated;

otherwise, use sanitizing wipes that contain alcohol or other antibacterial agents to thoroughly remove all dirt from your hands. Remember to pack out used wipes in a sealed plastic bag. Most are biodegradable, but some contain ingredients that could be harmful to the environment. Follow up with a hand sanitizing gel to ensure that all germs are killed. Carry a small bottle of hand sanitizer in your pocket and use it frequently: after bathroom breaks, before eating, and before cooking dinner. This cuts down on the risk of ingesting bacteria and other germs that can make you sick. It is not always sufficient to use sanitizing gel only; germs can survive underneath dirt and grime on the skin. Hot water typically is a rare wilderness commodity. But you can still get clean hands by substituting a germicidal rinse for hot water. Adequate hand sanitation can be achieved with a germicidal rinse and a cup or two of cold water. Ask your pharmacist to recommend a germicidal product used in hospitals. You can also get these products at hospital supply companies.

Always clean your hands before touching food. This is especially important if one person is doing the cooking for everybody in the group; infectious germs are often spread through the unsafe preparation and handling of food. The consequences can be disastrous if everybody in the group gets sick at the same time. Keep your fingernails short and clean.

- **Take care of your feet** – Keeping your feet clean and dry reduces the risk of blisters, and prevents bacterial and fungal growth on the skin. Bacteria and fungi thrive inside hot, sweaty hiking boots. Esure that your feet are clean before you put on your boots in the morning, and before you go to bed at night. Put on a clean pair of socks every morning. If you prefer sleeping with socks, pack a pair just for sleeping. Soak your feet whenever you stop at a river, creek or lake. Cleaning and drying your feet a couple of times a day reduces bacteria and fungi, and relieves hot spots before they can become blisters.

If water is plentiful, wash your socks and hang them out to dry overnight. Always make sure you have at least one dry pair for the next day, since socks won't always dry out completely overnight. Tie wet socks outside your backpack during the day. If water is not available, regularly clean your feet with antibacterial or alcohol wipes. Use foot powder to keep your feet dry and comfortable. If you are prone to athlete's foot or on an extended trip, use a product that contains an antifungal ingredient. Take off your boots and air your feet as often as you can. Keep your toenails short and clean.

- **Don't neglect dental hygiene** – It is important to maintain dental hygiene on the trail. Pack a travel-sized toothbrush, enough toothpaste and dental floss.
- **Be considerate** – Coughing, sneezing and blowing your nose spread your germs around. Always pack enough facial tissues or toilet paper to blow your nose and to protect others when you sneeze. Cover your mouth when you cough. Don't cough, sneeze or

blow your nose in the vicinity of food. Wash and/or sanitize your hands before handling food, before and after administering first aid, and after taking a toilet break. It is in your best interest to help keep others in your group healthy; in a backcountry emergency people have only one another to rely on for survival. Even under normal conditions, a sick member of the party becomes a liability to others and can very quickly spoil the trip for everybody.

- **Wash cooking and eating utensils after you have used them** – Use sufficient hot water and a good biodegradable dish soap to clean dishes. If it is not possible or practical to heat the water first, use cold water. Some soaps will work equally well in hot or cold water. Your best insurance against foodborne germs, however, is to sanitize your dishes and utensils after washing and rinsing. The simplest and most effective way is to soak them in a solution of one teaspoon of household bleach per litre of water for five minutes or more. I always carry a small plastic bottle of bleach in my backpack. You don't need much: 240 ml/8 fl. oz. is sufficient for a two-week trip, assuming you use one teaspoon three times per day. Take less for shorter outings. Chlorine bleach is also an excellent chemical to purify water with (see *Drinking Water*). No one should venture into the wilderness without at least a small bottle of bleach for emergency use. Ensure that the bottle seals tightly, and place it inside a strong sealable plastic bag to prevent damage to your clothes and gear.

If water is at a premium, use a small plastic spray bottle to spray the bleach solution onto clean dishes and utensils. Allow utensils to air dry, do not rinse or wipe them. Alternatively, use antibacterial or alcohol wipes to sanitize dishes and utensils after washing and rinsing them. If water for washing dishes is unavailable, use disposable plates and utensils, or pack food and drinks that can be consumed directly from their containers. Always pack out used plates, cups, packaging and other disposable items.

- **Keep flies and other insects away from your food and drinks** – or, as is usually the case on backpacking and other wilderness trips, keep your food away from insects and other animals.
- **Don't eat leftover food** – Leftovers result from cooking more food than we can eat. Storing uneaten food in the wilderness presents us with a difficult problem. Bacteria and many other germs thrive at temperatures between 4° C/40° F and 60° C/140° F and high levels of bacteria can be reached in food very quickly. Reheating cooked food, although it kills most bacteria, often leaves toxins produced by the bacteria. There may be sufficient toxins in even small quantities of food to cause serious diarrheal illness.

Your safest bet is to get rid of leftovers. Food waste can be buried, provided you bury it deep enough and a good distance from the camp. If campfires are permitted and safe in the area, dry food and small amounts of wet food can be burned effectively; large quantities of wet food usually congeal into a lump of

CAMPING & OUTDOORS

ash unless the fire is really hot. You can also scatter small amounts of food in remote areas as long as you do so well clear of your campsite, trails and surface water. Ideally, leftover food should be sealed in plastic bags and packed out.

- **Keep a safe distance from people who are coughing, sneezing, and anyone suffering from diarrhea or other illness** – Make sure that they wash their hands frequently and don't allow them to handle other people's food, or share utensils with others.

- **Pay attention to drinking water safety** – We need plenty of potable water every day; more so when we are active in the outdoors. Water helps us stay cool, digest our food, and keeps us alive. Drinking unsafe water can also kill us, or make us seriously ill. Never take a chance by drinking water that may not be safe. Most wilderness water sources in North America are unsafe to drink. The *Giardia* parasite is found in 90% of these waters. The symptoms of infection with this microbe include severe diarrhea, nausea and vomiting. Spring water can also be contaminated with *Giardia* and other parasites like *Cryptosporidium*. The safest thing to do is to bring your own water from home. However, it is sometimes necessary to use water from a wilderness source. Wilderness water must be treated to make it safe for drinking, brushing teeth, cooking or washing dishes. There are several methods for treating water found along the trail. These methods are discussed in detail in the *Drinking Water* chapter.

SURVIVAL OF THE CLEANEST

- ■ **Pit toilet pitfalls** – Pit toilets are a kind of necessary evil found at some wilderness campsites. They are convenient, especially after a long day's hiking or kayaking, and let's face it, we're just not made to squat on the ground. On the other hand, they can be filthy, smelly, infectious disease traps. In addition to protecting our own health, we also have to use pit toilets in such a way that we don't jeopardize other campers. There are a number of rules for safely using pit toilets:

  - Always keep the door closed. This will keep animals out of the facility.
  - Never touch the toilet door or latch with your bare hands. Just because a pit toilet stands out in the wilderness does *not* mean it's germ-free. On the contrary: toilet doorhandles and latches are virtually guaranteed to be contaminated with feces, urine and possibly even other body fluids. Millions of harmful germs thrive in these conditions. Most people do not clean or disinfect their hands after using a pit toilet. There usually is no running water provided, nor will you typically find hand sanitizer dispensers provided in a wilderness campsite. And far too few campers and backpackers bother to bring their own sanitizing gel or wipes. Pit toilets out in the woods are infrequently cleaned at best, some never.

    Know this: The doorhandle in that quaint little pit toilet out in the middle of nowhere is teeming with infectious germs that can cause any number of debilitating diseases. Just because there aren't other people around also does not indicate the absence of germs; germs can live for a long time in the kind of conditions provided

CAMPING & OUTDOORS

by a pit toilet. You can become infected with germs deposited on a latch many days earlier. Always use a paper towel, a thick wad of toilet paper or heavy duty facial tissue to protect your hands when opening or closing a pit toilet door – from the inside *and* the outside. It's not a bad idea to give the doorhandle and latch a quick spray with a disinfectant. Or you can wipe it down with a sanitizing wipe, or a paper towel soaked in a bleach solution. Definitely do this if you are staying in the site more than one day, or if you have young children in your party.

- Beware of the toilet seat! Follow the rules for using a public toilet described in *Public Washrooms*. In a nutshell: avoid sitting down if possible; if you have to sit down, cover and/or disinfect the seat surface. We always sanitize pit toilet seats and doorhandles when we get to a new campsite. It has become part of our routine for setting up camp. Disinfectant sprays and wipes both work fine.
- Do not use the pit toilet as a receptacle for garbage, this will attract wild animals, and some items can be harmful to the environment.
- Use your own toilet paper, even if some is provided. Who knows how long that roll has been sitting there, how many times it ended up on the floor or worse, or what insects have nested inside? Use antibacterial wipes in addition to toilet paper. You will not only feel cleaner and more comfortable; you'll also prevent getting a rash or infection.
- If there is lime powder or ashes provided, sprinkle some in the receptacle when you are finished. This will ensure that the waste matter is broken down faster, and it helps to control those nasty odours.

SURVIVAL OF THE CLEANEST

- ALWAYS clean your hands after using a pit toilet. If enough water is available, leave a container with water and liquid soap (preferably antibacterial) just outside the toilet. For additional protection, add chlorine bleach to the water, at the rate of one tablespoon of bleach per gallon of water, or about one teaspoon per litre. If water is limited, fill a small container with a strong disinfectant such as Dettol™ or Savlon™ to provide a one-stop cleaning setup. To use, dispense a small amount of the solution onto your hands, rub your hands together for about 30 seconds, shake off the excess and allow your hands to air dry. This is a very effective method for keeping hands sanitary in the field. It is even used by the military in some countries to prevent infectious disease outbreaks when troops are deployed for battle or other manoeuvres. An intravenous fluid (IV) bag filled with a disinfectant solution works extremely well for this purpose. It is small, lightweight and compactable, made of very durable plastic and the wheel mechanism used to regulate flow is perfect for dispensing the disinfectant solution.

  When no water can be spared for washing hands, use antibacterial wipes or hand sanitizer, preferably a combination of the two. Hand sanitizer gel on its own will not remove dirt and grime, and some germs may survive beneath the dirt. Antibacterial wipes do a good job of removing bacteria, but may not kill other germs like viruses and fungi. Wipes that contain alcohol in addition to other antibacterial agents are very effective.

- Flies, wasps and mosquitoes can be a problem around pit toilets in summer. Apply insect repellent to your clothes and exposed skin, and spray inside the facility to protect yourself against insect-borne infections.

CAMPING & OUTDOORS

▪ **Be careful with 'cat-holes'** – In areas where pit toilets are not provided, we have to use cat-holes. Cat-holes are shallow holes, dug a few inches deep and covered with a layer of soil after use. Disposing of human waste in the wilderness must be done with discretion and common sense. We have to ensure that we avoid contaminating the environment and making it unsafe for other people. One of the sources of *Giardia lamblia* in the wilderness is the careless disposal of human waste. Fecal-borne germs can infect us in several ways: direct contact with the feces, indirect contact with hands that have directly touched the feces, contact with insects that have contacted the feces, and drinking contaminated water. Take the following precautions to protect your health and that of your fellow campers, and to limit the impact on the environment:

- Human waste should be disposed of in a way that reduces the possibility of other people and animals discovering it. Pick a spot that is at least 70 metres/230 feet away from your campsite, and any trails or roads.
- A cat-hole 'kit' includes a backpacker's shovel, toilet paper, sanitary wipes and hand sanitizer gel. If you don't have a shovel, use a piece of wood or a flat rock to dig a hole; never dig with your hands.
- Always dispose of solid body wastes in a way that accelerates the decomposition process. Human feces is broken down to a harmless state by bacterial action in the presence of oxygen, moisture and heat. It is further sterilized by ultraviolet radiation from the sun. Choose a spot with maximum sunlight for faster decomposing.

SURVIVAL OF THE CLEANEST

Dig a hole 15 to 20 centimetres/6 to 8 inches deep into the soil. Use a stick to stir the solid waste into the soil to kick-start decomposition. Cover the hole with a layer of soil and disguise the spot to hide it from view.

- To prevent contaminating water in the area, cat-holes should be at least 70 metres/230 feet away from any water source.
- Use disposable sanitary wipes for proper hygiene. I strongly recommend using a good antibacterial brand.
- Wash or otherwise clean and disinfect your hands when you're finished. See the section on pit toilets above for detail.

■ **Don't share!** – People who share their water bottles, food or eating utensils are not doing anyone a favour, no matter how well-intentioned they are. Never share items like lip balm, towels, washcloths, toothbrushes, personal eating utensils or any toiletry items. Dispose of leftover food, energy bars or drinks and don't finish other people's meals or drinks.

■ **Keep insects at bay** – Insect bites and stings are not only annoying and painful; they can infect you with germs that will make you seriously ill. Always take the necessary precautions to protect against insect bites. See the *Insects* chapter for more information on this topic. Basic precautions include:

- Always wear protective clothing. Make sure that your neck, ankles and wrists are protected. Light-coloured clothing is less attractive to insects than dark clothing.
- Avoid using scented deodorants, sunscreen, lotions or perfume. Insects are attracted by these scents.

CAMPING & OUTDOORS

- Check your clothes regularly for insects, especially if you are in tick country.
- Keep your tent's insect screen closed at all times, and use a mosquito net to protect against mosquitoes and other flying insects. Spraying the screen or net with an insect repellent increases its effectiveness.
- When visiting an area with a large insect population, always use an insect repellent. Using chemical insect repellents is a must when you find yourself in mosquito, sand fly, or tick territory.

■ **Ensure that your hands are clean before gathering wild foods** like berries, mushrooms, mussels, etc. Use clean containers or plastic bags for collecting and storing harvested food.

■ **Disinfect your hands before administering first aid to anybody.** It is also a good idea to keep the outside of your first aid kit clean and germ-free. Disinfectant wipes work well for this task.

DRINKING WATER

We like to think of unsafe drinking water as strictly a problem in developing countries, of direct concern to us only when we travel. The reality is that any source of drinking water can be contaminated, and we should never assume that water is safe. While fatal outbreaks of waterborne disease are relatively rare in the industrialized world, tragedies like the deadly *E. coli* outbreak in Walkerton, Ontario do happen. In May of 2000, *E. coli* contamination of the town's water supply left seven people dead, and hundreds of others seriously ill. Worldwide, waterborne infectious diseases kill an estimated 40,000 people *every day*.

Bacteria and parasites are not the only contaminants in drinking water. Water can be contaminated with many different pollutants. Some pollutants occur naturally in the environment; others are caused by human activities.

Sources of Water Pollution

- *Micro-organisms* – Bacteria, viruses, parasites and other micro-organisms are sometimes found in water. Wells with water close to ground level are most at risk. Run-off water can accumulate germs, especially after flooding. These organisms can cause a variety of diarrheal and other illnesses.

- *Nitrates* – These contaminants are found in human and animal waste. Septic tanks, landfills, garbage dumps and farm animals are major sources of nitrate pollution. Fertilizers also increase nitrate levels. Nitrates can cause a serious condition in infants called 'blue baby' syndrome. This condition disrupts oxygen flow in the blood.
- *Animal Feeding Operations* – On these 'factory farms' thousands of animals are raised in a small area. The massive amounts of manure produced on these farms can pollute water supplies if not carefully managed.
- *Heavy Metals* – Mining, construction, farming and other activities that change the landscape can cause large amounts of heavy metals to be released into nearby groundwater. These metals pose a health risk if they are present at high levels in drinking water.
- *Fertilizers and Pesticides* – Fertilizers, pesticides and herbicides are widely used on farms, golf courses, lawns and in suburban gardens to promote plant growth, reduce insect damage and to control weeds. The chemicals in these products can contaminate groundwater. Many fertilizers contain nitrogen that can break down into harmful nitrates. Toxic chemicals used to treat buildings for termites and other pests can also pollute our drinking water.
- *Industrial Products and Wastes* – Many harmful chemicals are used widely in local business and

industry. These can become water pollutants if they are not managed properly. The most common sources of such problems are:

- Factories, industrial plants, and businesses such as gas stations and dry cleaners.
- Petroleum products, chemicals, and industrial waste products stored in underground storage tanks can end up in the groundwater if tanks and pipes leak.
- Landfills and garbage dumps have a wide variety of pollutants that can seep into groundwater.

■ *Household Wastes* – Improper disposal of many household products, including cleaning solvents, used motor oil, paint, soaps and detergents can contaminate our drinking water.

■ *Lead and Copper* – Household plumbing materials are the most common source of lead and copper in home drinking water. Corrosive water may cause metals in pipes or soldered joints to leach into tap water. Older plumbing materials are more likely to contaminate water. These metals are harmful even in relatively low concentrations.

Common pathogens found in drinking water sources:

Bacteria	**Viruses**	**Protozoa**
E. coli	Enterovirus	*Cryptosporidium*
Campylobacter	Hepatitis A	*Giardia*
Salmonella	Norovirus	
Shigella	Rotavirus	

Bottled Water

There is a growing concern among many people about chemicals and other pollutants in tap water. Most people also believe that bottled water is always safer to drink than municipal tap water. While this may be the case in some developing countries, there is no evidence to support this assumption in Canada, the USA and other industrialized countries in Europe and elsewhere. Varying levels of bacteria, viruses and other contaminants are found in most bottled water products sold for drinking. Bottled water is usually filtered or treated to remove most harmful organisms, but it is not sterile.

In fact, bottled water is quite often manufactured from municipal tap water. The water is filtered to lower its mineral content, and to remove chlorine, fluoride and other chemicals. By law, only products labeled as spring, mineral, or artesian well water have to come from a potable underground source, and not from a community water supply. And there is no guarantee that water from underground sources is not contaminated with parasites such as *Cryptosporidium* and *Giardia,* although water that comes from a protected well or a protected spring is less likely to contain parasites than water from unprotected sources, such as rivers and lakes.

Bottled water sold in Canada is described by federal health authorities as 'generally of good microbiological and chemical quality,' and 'as safe to consume as tap water from a microbiological quality and chemical safety standpoint.' That is their rather formal way of saying that bottled water is no safer than tap water.

Bottled Water Safety

Health Canada advises taking a number of precautions when using bottled water:

- Stick to bottled water that has either been distilled, ozonated, microfiltered, filtered by reverse osmosis or disinfected with ultraviolet light. These treatments eliminate harmful bacteria and other contaminants from the bottled water. Read labels carefully!
- Buy only sealed products. Carefully examine the bottle before you buy it. Don't buy bottled water if sediment or floating material is present.
- Report any bottles with broken seals or products with visible contaminants to the store manager and public health officials.
- Examine the bottle and label for the following: manufacturing date or code, best-before-date, chemical analysis (declaration of minerals), treatment (for example, ozonized, ozonated, etc.), company contact number, location and type of source water.
- To be effective against *Cryptosporidium* (crypto), one of these processing methods must be listed: reverse osmosis treated, distilled, filtered through an *absolute* one micron or smaller filter, or one micron absolute.
- Do not refill old bottles. It is preferable to buy newly manufactured bottled water.
- Do not share bottles. Pour the water into clean cups or glasses if more than one person is using the bottle.
- Refrigerate bottled water if possible, especially after opening the bottle.

DRINKING WATER

- If you can't refrigerate bottled water, store it in a cool, clean place away from heat and sunlight. Although manufacturers give bottled water a shelf life of two years, some health authorities recommend replacing it after one year.
- Use only *sterile* bottled water for babies and infants. Read the label to see if the water is sterile. When in doubt, boil the water before use.
- People with compromised immune systems should only buy sterile or disinfected bottled water, or boil bottled water before use.
- If you are concerned about chemical and bacterial content, contact the manufacturer. Most can be contacted via the phone numbers on the labels, by mail or e-mail.
- Never use bottled water to clean or store contact lenses. Use only those products intended for use with contact lenses.

Water Coolers

Water coolers are not self-cleaning. Never assume that a water cooler is clean. To ensure drinking water safety, follow these procedures provided by Health Canada for cleaning your water cooler and replacing the bottle:

Cleaning

- Clean water coolers with every bottle change.
- Unplug the cord from the electrical outlet.

- Remove the empty bottle.
- Drain the water from the stainless steel reservoir through the faucet/s.
- Prepare a disinfecting solution by adding one tablespoon (15 ml) household bleach to one gallon/3.8 litres of water. Some companies recommend using a solution of one part vinegar to three parts water to clean the reservoir of scale before cleaning it with bleach.
- Wash the reservoir thoroughly with the bleach solution and let it stand for no less than two minutes (to be effective) and no more than five minutes (to prevent corrosion).
- Drain the bleach solution from the reservoir through the faucet/s.
- Rinse the reservoir thoroughly with clean tap water, draining the water through the faucet/s, to remove all traces of the bleach solution.
- Remove the drip tray and screen and wash them in dish detergent.
- Rinse the drip tray and screen thoroughly in clean tap water and replace them on the cooler.
- Use water coolers that filter the air that enters the bottle as the water level lowers.

Replacing the Bottle

- Wash your hands before handling the bottle. If you choose to use clean protective gloves (latex or vinyl), discard or disinfect them after each use.

DRINKING WATER

- Wipe the top and neck of the new bottle with a paper towel dipped in a household bleach solution (one tablespoon of bleach in one gallon of water). Rubbing alcohol may also be used, but must be completely evaporated before placing the bottle in the cooler.
- Remove the seal and place the bottle on the cooler.

Treating Water

Boiling

Boiling is the most reliable method to make water safe for drinking. Water should be kept at boiling point for at least one minute and allowed to cool to room temperature. Do not add ice. This procedure will kill bacteria and parasites at all altitudes and viruses at low altitudes. To kill viruses at altitudes above 2,000 m/6,562 ft, water should be boiled for at least three minutes, or chemically disinfected *after* the water has boiled for one minute. Add a pinch of salt for each litre/quart of boiled water or pour the water several times from one clean container to another to improve the taste.

It's a good idea to keep a small backpacker stove and a pot for boiling water in your emergency kit at home and in your vehicle.

Chemical Purification

Chemical disinfection with *iodine* or *chlorine* is an alternative method of water treatment when it is not feasible to boil water. However, this method cannot always be relied on to kill *Cryptosporidium* and *Giardia* parasites.

SURVIVAL OF THE CLEANEST

Two methods for disinfecting water with *iodine* are the use of iodine tablets and tincture of iodine. Iodine tablets are available from pharmacies and sporting goods stores. Follow the manufacturer's instructions. Use one tablet for each litre/quart of water if the instructions are missing. If the water is cloudy, the number of tablets used should be doubled; if the water is extremely cold (below 5° C/ 41° F), it should be warmed up if possible, and the recommended contact time should be doubled to achieve reliable disinfection.

Tincture of iodine, available at any drug store and found in most medicine chests and first aid kits, can also be used to disinfect water. Add five drops of tincture of iodine to each litre/quart of clear water. Cloudy water requires at least ten drops per litre/quart of water. Let the solution stand for 30 minutes or longer. Cloudy water should be filtered or strained through a clean cloth to remove sediment or floating matter, and then treated with iodine. Iodine tablets have a shelf life of about three months, after which they should be replaced.

Chlorine, in liquid or tablet form, can also be used for chemical disinfection. However, its germicidal activity varies greatly with the pH, temperature and organic content of the water. This can cause inconsistent levels of purification in some types of water. Filtration or microfiltration of water before chlorine treatment can improve the effectiveness of chlorine disinfection. Chlorine tablets are available from drug stores and stores that sell camping and other outdoor equipment. Follow the manufacturer's instructions for use. If instructions are not available, use one tablet for each litre/quart of water.

DRINKING WATER

Household (chlorine) bleach may also be used to purify water. Add two drops for each litre/quart of water; four drops per litre/quart if the water is cloudy or very cold. Mix the treated water well, and let it stand, covered, for at least 30 minutes. If you use a bleach product with less than four percent of available chlorine (check the label), increase the treatment to ten drops per litre/quart for clear water; 20 drops for cloudy or cold water. The same applies if the chlorine concentration is unknown.

To purify larger quantities of water, add regular household bleach (five percent chlorine) at the rate of four drops per gallon of water. For example, treating ten gallons of water will require 40 drops of bleach. Cover and let it stand for at least two hours. The effectiveness of treating water with bleach also depends on the time the treated water is allowed to stand before use. The longer you can let it stand, the safer the water will be.

Treating water with chlorine bleach is not very effective against *Giardia* or *Cryptosporidium* parasites. Boiling is the best way to remove these parasites from your drinking water.

Chemically treated water is intended for short-term use only. If iodine-disinfected water is the only water available, it should not be used for more than a few weeks. Keep iodine purification tablets and a small plastic bottle of household bleach in your emergency kit.

*****

SURVIVAL OF THE CLEANEST

Water Filters

Filtering Tap Water:

Many different types of water filters are available for home use. They range from activated charcoal filters that do little more than remove chlorine and other chemicals from water, to reverse osmosis filtration systems that produce water that is practically 100% pure. Filters collect micro-organisms and other contaminants from water. The quality of tap water available in your area will determine what kind of filter you need to use. If, like most people in Canada and the US, you live in a city or town with safe municipal water, a simple charcoal filter to remove chlorine and improve the water's taste may suffice. On the other hand, if you get your water from a well, river or lake, you will require a filtration system that can remove bacteria, viruses, protozoa like *Cryptosporidium*, and other contaminants.

Not all available home water filters will remove *Cryptosporidium*. Some filter designs are more suitable for removal of *Cryptosporidium* than others. Filters that use reverse osmosis will remove *Cryptosporidium*. Microfilters designed to remove particles less than or equal to one micron in diameter also provide protection against this parasite. There are two types of microfilters: *absolute one micron* filters and *nominal one micron* filters. Absolute one micron filters will consistently remove *Cryptosporidium*. Some nominal one micron filters will allow 20% to 30% of one micron particles to pass through. It is important to understand what your filter's capabilities and limitations are. Read the label and

DRINKING WATER

instructions carefully. When in doubt, always boil water before drinking. Filters that are designed to remove *Cryptosporidium* and *Giardia* will always include one of the following four treatments on the label:

- Reverse osmosis.
- Absolute pore size of one micron or smaller.
- Tested and certified by NSF Standard 53 or NSF Standard 58 for cyst *removal*.
- Tested and certified by NSF Standard 53 or NSF Standard 58 for cyst *reduction*.

Filters may not remove *Cryptosporidium* if labeled only with these words:

- Nominal pore size of ≤ one micron.
- One micron filter.
- Effective against *Giardia*.
- Effective against parasites.
- Carbon filter.
- Water purifier.
- EPA approved (EPA does not approve or test filters).
- EPA registered (EPA does not register filters for crypto removal).
- Activated carbon.
- Removes chlorine.
- Ultraviolet light.
- Pentiodide resins.
- Water softener.

Anyone changing filter cartridges should wear gloves and wash their hands afterwards. People who are HIV positive or immune impaired should never change filter cartridges. Filters may not remove bacteria, viruses and protozoa as effectively as boiling; even good brands of filters can have manufacturing flaws that allow some micro-organisms to pass through the filter. Poor filter maintenance or failing to replace filter cartridges as recommended by the manufacturer can also result in unsafe drinking water.

Proper selection, operation, care and maintenance of water filters are essential to producing safe water. The manufacturer's instructions should be followed. NSF International, an independent testing company, tests and certifies water filters for their ability to remove protozoa, but not for their ability to remove bacteria or viruses.

Portable Filters:

Portable filters will provide different levels of protection against microbes. Reverse osmosis filters provide protection against viruses, bacteria, and protozoa, but they are expensive, are larger than most filters used by backpackers, and the small pores on this type of filter are rapidly clogged by muddy or cloudy water.

Microfilters with pore sizes in the one to three micron range can remove bacteria and protozoa from drinking water, but they do not remove viruses. To kill viruses, people using microstrainer filters should disinfect the water with iodine or chlorine after filtration. Microfilters that incorporate iodine resins are effective against bacteria, protozoa and most viruses, and offer the convenience of one-step treatment. Purifier bottles are useful and practical for producing smaller quantities of safe drinking water in the backcountry or when traveling. They offer a lightweight, self-contained water purification system tailored for individual use. Purifier bottles utilize iodine-impregnated microfilters that remove or kill most bacteria, viruses and protozoa in the water. Simply fill the bottle, replace the filter and cap, squeeze and drink. Microfilter bottles are less expensive and will provide protection against bacteria and protozoa. To kill viruses, the water has to be purified with chlorine or iodine, or boiled before drinking.

A word of caution: Many portable filters and purifiers will *not* remove all *Cryptosporidium* and *Giardia* parasites from water. Boiling is the best method for eliminating these organisms.

Home Distillers

You can remove crypto and other germs from your water with a home distiller. Distillers work by evaporating and condensing water, the same way rain water is formed. Distilled water is very pure and virtually free of contaminants. If you use a distiller, you need to store your water as recommended for storing purified water.

Ultraviolet Purification

Ultraviolet light has been used to purify water in municipal water treatment facilities, hospitals and water bottling plants for over 60 years. Home-use ultraviolet purifiers have been available for a number of years and are becoming more popular, with good reason.

Ultraviolet purifiers utilize a germicidal ultraviolet lamp that produces radiation lethal to bacteria, viruses, protozoa and other micro-organisms present in water. They offer rapid water treatment without the use of heat or chemicals. Ultraviolet light deactivates the DNA of bacteria, viruses, protozoa and other pathogens. This destroys their ability to multiply and cause disease.

One of the main benefits of ultraviolet purification technology is its non-chemical approach to disinfection. In this method of disinfection, nothing is added to the water, which makes the process simple, inexpensive and doesn't alter the taste of the water.

Ultraviolet purifiers are available for many different applications: under-sink installations for home use, water vending machines, aircraft, boats, water wells, hot tubs, schools, hotels, ice-making machines and others.

Home purification systems that combine a reverse osmosis filter with ultraviolet treatment offer a very high level of protection and produce water that is, for all intents and purposes, 100% pure.

Portable Ultraviolet Purifiers

At the time of writing, there is at least one product available that employs ultraviolet technology in a practical, portable design for purifying water anywhere. Other products are sure to follow. The product currently on the market is about the size of an electric toothbrush and uses ultraviolet light to destroy microbes in small volumes of water. Clear water from any source can be sterilized by destroying viruses, bacteria and protozoa, including *Giardia* and *Cryptosporidium*, in a few seconds.

It will not remove sediment, metals or chemicals from water, or do anything to improve the taste. It should therefore only be used for purifying clear or filtered water. I expect to see many new products on the market that utilize ultraviolet technology.

Storing Water

Water does not have an unlimited shelf life. Purified water should preferably be refrigerated or, at least, stored in a cool, clean place away from heat and direct sunlight. Purified water or store-bought bottled water should not be stored for more than one year.

Water can only be as clean as the container it is stored in. Sterilize containers with boiling water, a chlorine solution or other food-safe sanitizers before filling. Use strong containers that seal tightly. Reusable water bottles should be washed and sanitized before each refill.

Private Well Resources

Between 14 and 15 million households in the United States, and an estimated 25% of Canadian households rely on private wells for drinking water.

As a rule, groundwater is naturally clean and safe for domestic use. The overlying soil acts as a filter to keep groundwater free from disease-causing micro-organisms and other contaminants. There are, unfortunately, many exceptions to the rule. Wells can become contaminated due to various factors, such as improper location, incorrect installation of well casings or caps, breaks in the casing, or when contaminated surface water enters the well.

If you have a private well, it is important to know when to test and how to maintain your well properly to protect your family's health. The following should be considered in protecting your drinking water and maintaining your well:

- Distance of the well from sources of human wastes such as septic systems.
- Mining, farming or industrial activities in the area that can affect the quality of water in the well.
- Proximity of animal feedlots or manure spreading.
- The types of soil and underlying rocks.
- Behaviour of surface water: does water flow easily or collect on the surface?
- Required minimum depth to avoid seasonal changes in groundwater supply.
- The age of the well, its pump, and other parts.
- Protecting the water distribution system from cross connections and backflow.

Basic Precautions

There are six basic steps to ensure the safety of a well:

- Identify potential problem sources.
- Talk with local experts.

DRINKING WATER

- Have your water tested periodically.
- Learn how to interpret the test results, or consult with an expert to explain them to you.
- Set a regular maintenance schedule for your well; stick to the schedule and keep accurate records.
- Fix any problems without delay.

Testing Well Water

Well water should be tested every year for total coliform bacteria, nitrates, total dissolved solids and pH levels. If there is a risk of other contaminants, test for these also.

Before taking a sample, contact the laboratory that will perform your tests for instructions and sampling bottles. Follow their instructions carefully.

It is important to test well water after replacing or repairing any part of the well system (piping, pump, or the well itself). Also test if you notice a change in your water's appearance, taste, or smell.

HYGIENE IN THE HOME

Protecting your home against germs requires more than just vacuuming, dusting and washing the floors. While these activities are important, there are other hazards you need to be aware of and guard against.

The germs that can contaminate our homes come from two main sources. There are germs that occur naturally in our homes, and then there are those germs we pick up in other places and bring into the house with us. We will refer to them as *naturally occurring* and *introduced germs* respectively.

Naturally Occurring Germs

Naturally occurring germs are found in many environments, including in our homes. In sanitary, clean conditions they usually don't pose a huge risk to our health. Dirty and unsanitary conditions, on the other hand, provide the perfect environment for germs to live, multiply and spread. If we don't clean and disinfect the high-risk areas in our homes frequently, we gamble with our families' health.

It is important to know where the 'hot zones' or high-risk areas in our homes are. These areas should be

HYGIENE IN THE HOME

routinely cleaned and correctly disinfected to reduce the opportunity for germs to multiply and spread. Think of it as a war strategy; if you destroy the enemy's infrastructure, you stand a better chance of winning the war.

There are four proven methods for destroying germs in the home:

- **Cleaning** – Washing an object or surface with detergent and hot water is often sufficient to remove germs. Scrub it vigorously to loosen the dirt and germs, and then rinse it thoroughly with clean water. This method is effective for household dishes, floors, walls, and keeping hands germ-free.
- **Disinfecting** – Disinfectants should be used where surfaces or objects cannot be washed and rinsed effectively, and where there is an increased risk of infection. Kitchen counters and floors, toilets, doorhandles, pet bedding areas, bathtubs, showers, garbage cans, bathroom floors and kitchen sinks should be disinfected regularly.
- **Drying** – Most germs cannot survive in a clean, dry environment. Wet kitchen and bathroom surfaces, damp cleaning cloths, wet towels and dirty mops can all harbour and spread germs around the house.
- **Heating** – As a rule, higher temperatures will kill more germs. Launder clothes, towels, cleaning cloths, linen and pet bedding at high temperatures of at least 60°C/140° F to destroy germs. Cook food thoroughly to reduce the germs present in the food to a level that is safe to eat. Wash dishes in hot water.

SURVIVAL OF THE CLEANEST

While we should keep every part of our home clean and germ-free, there are several areas that warrant closer attention. These areas are the kitchen, bathrooms, dining room, TV room, any other rooms where food or snacks are consumed, bedding and feeding areas for pets, doorhandles, any deck or outside areas where food is prepared or served, laundry room, garbage cans, and any areas that are damp or not well-ventilated, such as the basement.

Cleaning and disinfecting are not the same thing. In some cases, cleaning with soap and water is adequate. It removes dirt and most of the germs. Disinfecting provides an extra margin of safety. This is because disinfectants, including solutions of household bleach, have ingredients that destroy bacteria and other germs. While surfaces may look clean, many infectious germs may be lurking around. Given the right conditions some germs can live on surfaces for hours and even for days.

Kitchen Hygiene

The kitchen is one of the most dangerous places in the house, mainly because of the infectious bacteria that are found in raw food such as chicken, red meat and fish. Also, there is an opportunity for germs to be passed on to other people because that is where food is prepared.

Raw meat and poultry, eggs, fish and unwashed fruit and vegetables can all carry germs. Thoroughly cooking food and maintaining scrupulous kitchen hygiene are the primary ways to prevent food poisoning. For additional information and advice see the *Food Safety* chapter.

HYGIENE IN THE HOME

Bacteria can multiply quickly in moist environments, such as in food left to stand at room temperature or in damp cleaning cloths.

- Always wash your hands before preparing food and immediately after handling raw foods, especially red meat, poultry and seafood.
- Use a disposable paper towel to dry your hands.
- Make sure that kitchen work surfaces are sanitized immediately before use. Use a quality disinfectant.
- Regularly disinfect objects that you frequently touch with your hands, such as door and cupboard handles, taps and the wastebin.
- Routinely clean and disinfect the fridge, microwave, cupboards, and any other surfaces that come into frequent contact with food.
- Use a garbage bin with a lid to prevent access by pets, rodents and insects.
- Empty, clean and disinfect garbage bins often.
- Do not allow pets in the kitchen.
- Wear clean clothes or a clean apron when handling, preparing or serving food.

Bathroom Hygiene

Another danger zone in the home is the bathroom. Regularly cleaning and disinfecting the bathroom eliminates odours and helps to prevent the spread of germs when someone in the house has a diarrheal or other contagious illness. The greatest risk of infection in the bathroom comes from surfaces we frequently touch: toilet flushing handles, toilet seats, taps and doorknobs. You should regularly disinfect these surfaces. Disposable cleaning cloths or wipes are easy to use and hygienic.

Follow these guidelines to keep your bathrooms clean and safe:

- Clean and disinfect toilet bowls frequently to remove dirt and grime that can shelter germs and cause bad odours. Use a suitable toilet bowl cleaning product. Rinse and disinfect the toilet brush after use.
- Clean up any spills immediately and disinfect the contaminated surfaces. Disposable paper towels or disinfectant wipes are convenient to use for this task.
- Wash out bathtubs and rinse sinks after each use. Clean and disinfect them often with a product that is formulated to effectively remove lime scale, soap scum and germs. Disinfect shower stalls regularly.
- Showerheads can harbour germs. If the shower hasn't been used for a while, let the hot water run on full power for two minutes to flush out any germs before taking a shower.
- Clean and disinfect shower curtains with a suitable product or launder them in the washing machine. Dry in the dryer at the highest temperature setting.
- Store personal items, such as toothbrushes, in a closed cabinet or container to protect them from airborne germs in the bathroom. Rinse them after each use and store them dry. Never share personal items.
- Launder and replace towels frequently.

HYGIENE IN THE HOME

- Launder bathroom floor mats regularly.
- Keep the bathroom clean, dry and well-ventilated to prevent the growth of mold and to avoid attracting flies and other pests.
- Clean and disinfect diaper pails and changing tables for babies at least daily.
- Wash your hands thoroughly after using the toilet and after cleaning the bathroom.
- Keep the cover closed when flushing the toilet to contain the germ-contaminated aerosol created by flushing.

Floors, Furniture and Household Surfaces

Washing hard surface floors with a detergent and warm water will remove dust, dirt, germs and mold growth. Vacuuming carpets and upholstered furniture removes dust, dust mites, pet hair and other debris. You should always disinfect surfaces that have been contaminated by food spills, pet accidents or human body fluids. Hard surface floors are preferable in bathrooms and kitchens; they are easier to keep clean and they do not collect dirt and debris the way carpets do.

The best way to routinely clean and disinfect surfaces is described below. By following these simple steps, you get the maximum benefit for your cleaning efforts, and the most protection for your family.

- Choose appropriate cleaning products. Look for products that contain chlorine bleach. Chlorine or household bleach is a very effective disinfectant.

SURVIVAL OF THE CLEANEST

Follow the directions on the cleaning product labels and read the safety precautions as well. Antibacterial hand soaps and dish washing liquids don't disinfect hard surfaces like countertops, sinks and faucets.

- Clean food and pet spills immediately after they happen. This will reduce the opportunity for germ growth, and it is usually easier to get stains out if you attend to them right away.
- Use disposable paper towels to remove spills of body fluids, then clean and disinfect the surface.
- To disinfect, first clean the surface thoroughly with soap and water or another cleaner. After cleaning, apply the disinfectant to the area, and let it stand for a few minutes or longer. Follow the manufacturer's instructions. This keeps the germs in contact with the disinfectant longer. Wipe the surface with paper towels or disposable wipes.
- If you are cleaning up body fluids such as blood, vomit, or feces, you should wear rubber gloves, particularly if you have cuts or scratches on your hands or if a family member has HIV/AIDS, hepatitis B, or another bloodborne disease. It is also a good idea to clean *and* disinfect surfaces when someone in the house is sick.
- If you use a mop and bucket, disinfect them with a chlorine bleach solution after each use and store them in a dry place.
- Moisten hard furniture surfaces before wiping them to minimize airborne dust and debris.

HYGIENE IN THE HOME

- To prevent the growth of mold and fungi, clean and disinfect tiled walls and other hard surfaces where moisture is likely to collect.
- Do not use bleach products on carpets, wooden surfaces or in unventilated areas.
- Remember to wash your hands after doing cleaning chores around the house.
- Before going to bed or before leaving the house, use disinfecting wipes to wipe down kitchen counters and appliances, so your kitchen is clean when you return home from work or get up in the morning.
- Store cleaners and disinfectants out of the reach of children and pets.
- Even if you use gloves, wash your hands thoroughly after cleaning or disinfecting surfaces.
- Regularly vacuum carpets and upholstery, more often if you have pets or small children. To remove odours, sprinkle baking soda, or a carpet deodorizer formulated with baking soda, on carpets and upholstery, wait 15 minutes, then vacuum.
- Regularly clean and disinfect telephones, computer keyboards and mice, remote controls, game consoles, doorhandles (including fridge, oven and cupboard doorhandles), and other frequently handled objects. Use disinfectant wipes or paper towels moistened with a disinfectant.

*****

SURVIVAL OF THE CLEANEST

Garbage Cans

It is easy to forget that garbage is first and foremost a public health issue. We worry so little about our trash that we keep it in our homes in transfer stations we euphemistically call wastebins.

Garbage cans are germ traps. All the germs that can be found in decaying food waste and other discarded organic matter are found in indoor and outdoor bins. These include several of the bacteria that can cause food poisoning, such as *E. coli, Listeria monocytogenes* and *Campylobacter jejuni*.

If cans are left open they attract flies, cockroaches, rats and other pests that spread disease. Cans and bins that are not regularly emptied become the source of unpleasant smells.

To reduce your family's exposure to the health risks posed by garbage, always take the following practical precautions:

- Invest in good, strong garbage bins with tight-fitting lids.
- Containerize garbage to discourage flies, rats and other pests.
- Wrap and place garbage and other organic wastes in sealed plastic garbage bags. Place these bags in a garbage can that is cleaned on a regular basis.
- Put your garbage out for pick-up on the morning of your scheduled pick-up.
- If you have more garbage than your cans can hold, you may be able to purchase tags or extra bags from

HYGIENE IN THE HOME

your service provider for occasional excesses. If you have regular excess garbage you must arrange for increased service.

- Always use refuse bags and tie them up before removing to avoid garbage spilling into the can.
- Regularly clean bins with hot water and a strong household detergent, and then disinfect them with a chlorine bleach solution.
- Clean and disinfect outside cans after each collection day. Clean and disinfect them inside and outside; pay special attention to the lid and handles.
- Don't place garbage cans too close to the house.

Recycling

Food and drink containers should be cleaned thoroughly before they are set aside for recycling.

Sandboxes

Children's sandboxes are not exempt from potential infection problems. Cats and other animals often use sandboxes as toilets. Disease-causing germs in their feces can be passed on to children when they play in the sand or to pets that can spread the germs indoors. Several diseases, including gastroenteritis and ringworm, are spread in this way.

There are a number of steps you can take to protect your children from sandbox infections:

- Rake the sand at least once a week to remove animal droppings and other debris.

- If you find animal waste or other contaminants, wash the sand with water. Let it dry before allowing the children back into the sandbox.
- Always cover the sandbox when it's not in use, but make sure you air it once in a while.
- Replace the sand every year, or if you suspect the sand might be contaminated.
- Do not allow children to eat or drink while playing in the sandbox.
- Ensure that children wash their hands after spending time in the sandbox.

Useful tip: A large built-in sandbox can be difficult to keep clean. Consider buying a portable plastic children's splash pool. Fill it with sand from a hardware store, which can be thrown out at the end of summer. Clam-type pools come with a plastic cover, which will keep animals out.

Airborne Germs

There are a number of things we can do to effectively reduce airborne germs in the home:

- The most obvious is to teach children (and sometimes adults) to cover their mouths and noses every time they cough or sneeze. This simple precaution will dramatically decrease the aerosolized viruses and bacteria we inhale in the home.
- Good housekeeping and household hygiene also play an important role in keeping the air safe to breathe. Clean, disinfected surfaces mean fewer germs that

can become airborne. Clean carpets and furniture mean less dust and other debris that can carry germs aloft. Clean kitchens and bathrooms don't produce bacteria and mold that can end up in our airways.
- Keep the home well-ventilated. Open windows when the weather permits and make sure bathroom and kitchen ventilation fans are clean and in good working condition.
- Heating and air conditioning ducts are major sources of airborne germs in many homes. Bacteria, mold and viruses can find a foothold in the dust, hair and other particles that collect in ducts. Regular, professional cleaning of ducts is a good investment in your own and your family's health.
- Many aerosol air cleaners and fresheners contain disinfectants that kill germs in the air. Products that contain ethyl alcohol or phenol will effectively reduce airborne bacteria, fungi and viruses in the home. *A word of caution:* Some people may be sensitive to the active ingredients in air disinfectants. Always follow the manufacturer's instructions and use caution around young children, pregnant women or people who suffer from asthma.
- High-efficiency particulate-arresting (HEPA) filters, available at discount drug stores, can remove pollen, dust, animal dander and some bacteria and viruses from the air. They are very effective at preventing symptoms for those who suffer from allergies, but can also decrease respiratory infections for everyone. Houseplants can also help to purify the air.

Introduced Germs

The danger of introduced germs is overlooked by many people. These are the potentially harmful microbes we collect on our hands, clothes and other items while we are at work, out shopping, dining out, visiting friends, waiting at the clinic or any other place we visit. These germs can quickly find a foothold and spread in our homes if we do not take the necessary precautions to avoid contamination. It is important to be aware of and to understand these threats to our health, and to know which steps to take to prevent germs from coming into, and spreading throughout the home. We have to also recognize those situations where contamination cannot be avoided entirely, and we have to know which actions to take to contain and eliminate the contamination before it can infect anyone in the household.

Germs can infiltrate our homes via contaminated hands, clothes, footwear, guests, pets, insects, rodents, food items, and other contaminated objects.

Hands

Our hands are the biggest culprits for bringing germs into the home. Any object or surface we touch at work, at the mall, at school, riding the bus, every place we visit, and every facility we use, is a potential carrier of harmful bacteria, viruses or fungi that can be transferred onto our hands. We deposit these germs onto any surface we touch at home where they can infect others in the household.

HYGIENE IN THE HOME

Thoroughly wash your hands immediately after you get home. Do this before you touch anything or anyone in the house. Don't even pet the dog or cat before washing your hands. The germs will happily live and multiply on the pet, and you or another family member will get them back with interest. This goes for everybody returning home from the outside.

Use a paper towel, toilet paper or your forearms to open and close faucets, otherwise you will contaminate them. Consider installing touchless faucets in your bathrooms. They are inexpensive, easy to install and fit standard bathroom and kitchen plumbing. A touchless faucet has a motion sensor that opens a valve, allowing the water to run for a few seconds when you hold your hands underneath it. As an added bonus, touchless faucets conserve water because they automatically close after a few seconds. This stops water from pouring down the drain unnecessarily while you scrub your hands.

The ideal solution is to have a place to wash your hands outside the house, or right by the door inside the house. The ultimate solution is an outdoor setup with hot water, touchless faucets, liquid soap dispenser and a motion-activated paper towel dispenser.

If these options are not practical or affordable, a quick, inexpensive solution is to mount a liquid soap dispenser on the wall next to an outside tap. Fill it with a good antibacterial soap, add a paper towel roll, and you have a perfectly workable setup for keeping hands clean before entering the house. You will find it equally useful when gardening, barbecuing, working on a vehicle, playing with the pets or doing anything outside the house that leaves your hands dirty.

Washing your hands first, before doing or touching anything inside the home, is a minor change to make in your routine. It goes a long way towards safeguarding your home against introduced germs.

Clothes and Footwear

The next big culprits for collecting and bringing germs into our homes are our clothes and shoes. Remove shoes and outer clothing, like jackets or sweaters, before or immediately after entering the house. Have a designated area by the door for leaving shoes and hanging jackets and coats. Never walk into the house with your shoes on. Not even when you're in a hurry. Consider for a moment all the places you have walked, and all the nasty dirt your shoes came into contact with. Remember the sticky floor at that foul-smelling public washroom you visited a few hours earlier?

Change your pants or dress as soon as possible after getting home; definitely before you sit down or prepare food. Washable clothing should go in the wash right away. Dry-clean only items should be cleaned often. Wash or dry-clean jackets and coats regularly.

Laundry Tips:

Correctly laundering clothing kills germs and drastically reduces the risk of infection.

- Washing clothes at high temperatures (at least 60°C/140° F) will destroy most germs.

HYGIENE IN THE HOME

- For fabrics that should be washed in cold water, add a laundry disinfectant to the washing water, or use a detergent that contains bleach to ensure that all germs are destroyed.
- Read the manufacturer's instructions for operating your washing machine.
- Use suitable cleaning products that will remove organic matter, such as blood, which can harbour all manner of germs.
- Before laundering heavily soiled items (for example washable diapers), dispose of any solid waste into the toilet, not the sink.
- Regularly disinfect the washing machine by adding a cup of bleach and running the rinse cycle.
- Keep dirty laundry away from food and food preparation areas.
- Launder kitchen cloths and towels separately from clothes and bed linen.
- Wash your hands thoroughly after handling dirty or wet laundry.
- Dry your washing as soon as laundering is complete. Germs and nasty odours can build up very quickly in damp laundry left inside a washing machine.

Food

Food items, especially raw meat, poultry and seafood, are major carriers of germs. Many raw foods contain natural bacteria that will grow in unsanitary conditions. Food or food packaging can also be contaminated by other foods or sources. Always exercise caution when handling food products. Follow the guidelines in the chapter on *Food Safety* for safely handling and storing perishable food products.

Wipe and disinfect the outside of meat, seafood and poultry packaging, and rinse dairy containers before storing them in the refrigerator. Ensure that there are no leaks in any of the packaging, and place raw food items in separate containers or plastic bags to avoid contact with other food or beverages in the fridge. Store raw meat, seafood and poultry products on a tray or on the bottom shelf to prevent any leaking juices from dripping onto other food or containers in the fridge.

Clean and disinfect all surfaces where raw food products were unpacked or handled. Contaminated food and food packaging can rightfully be regarded as the Trojan horses of the germ world.

Toiletries and Non-food Items

Toiletries and other non-food items can also become contaminated when people handle them in the store or at the checkout counter. Always assume that the outer packaging of any store-bought item has some level of germ contamination. Immediately remove and discard the outer packaging of your purchases. Disinfect items without removable outer packaging before using or storing them. Wash new clothes before wearing them.

Disinfect the counter or tabletop where you have unpacked your shopping bags. Remember to wash your hands once everything has been unpacked and cleaned.

HYGIENE IN THE HOME

Pets in the Home

Animals, like people, carry germs in and on their bodies. However, unlike (most of) us, animals pay no attention to where they deposit their germs. Keeping pets poses additional infection risks.

If you have pets, any areas of the house they have access to should be cleaned and disinfected frequently. If possible, limit their access to a specific area in the house. This makes it easier to keep clean and reduces the chance of your pets spreading germs around the house. Always use household bleach or a cleaner containing bleach when cleaning your pets' sleeping and feeding areas. In addition to hosting bacteria and viruses, dogs and cats are carriers of fungi and parasites, which are tough to kill with other cleaners.

Dogs are notorious for dragging dirt and germs into the house. They run through mud, muck and the waste left behind by other dogs. Some dogs have a weakness for rolling in anything that smells really rotten, the more unwholesome the better. Bad odours are caused by bacteria that your dog deposits all over your floors, carpets and furniture.

Always clean and disinfect dogs' feet before they are allowed inside the house. I recommend a quick two-step process to ensure that your dog's feet are clean and germ-free. First, give the dog's feet a thorough rinse with the garden hose. Pay special attention to the pads and the areas between the toes. Remove any debris matted in the hair. Next, disinfect the feet with a dog-friendly disinfectant solution. You can pour the solution into a plastic container that is deep enough to immerse the dog's foot and about two inches of the leg. Soak the feet for at least 15 seconds each. Alternatively, use a spray bottle to give the feet a good soaking with the disinfectant. Do not rinse after disinfecting; allow the disinfectant to dry on the dog's feet. Contain the dog in an area that can be easily cleaned afterwards.

If you live in an apartment or condo where an outside garden hose is not available, use a plastic tub or small bucket to wash the dog's feet and follow one of the disinfection options described above.

If your dog got dirty during the walk, or rolled in mud or worse, wash it properly before allowing access into the house. Do not wash your dog in the bathtub. Use a suitably sized plastic tub and wash the dog outside if at all possible. If you can't wash the dog outside, due to cold or wet weather, or if you don't have a garden, deck or balcony, wash the dog in a plastic tub inside the house, not in the bathtub.

Cats tend to be more hygienic and are usually a bit more discriminating about what they step or roll in. But, if you do have a cat with a hygiene problem, wash it often and clean and disinfect its feet.

In addition to following the basic, common sense rules described above, exotic pet owners should ensure that they have all the correct information about caring for and cleaning their exotic mammal or reptile. If you are thinking about keeping an exotic pet, bear in mind that exotic animals can be carriers of exotic, and potentially deadly viruses, bacteria, fungi or parasites. I do not recommend keeping exotic animals as pets.

HYGIENE IN THE HOME

General Pet Hygiene Tips:

- Take sick pets to a vet without delay.
- Wash your hands thoroughly after touching pets or handling food bowls and bedding.
- Pets should have their own food bowls and utensils.
- Wash and disinfect their food and water bowls daily. Do not wash them with household dishes.
- Immediately clean and disinfect any surface that has been contaminated with animal excretions. Remember to wash your hands!
- Never allow your pets onto food preparation surfaces or into food preparation areas.
- Regularly clean and disinfect the feeding areas used by your pets.
- Don't clean pet cages and tanks in the kitchen sink. Use a bucket or plastic tub instead.
- Do not let pets share your plate or lick your face.

For more information please see the next chapter, *Pets & Wild Animals*.

Insects and Rodents

Insects and rodents carry germs in and on their bodies. They can transmit their germs to us through direct contact, such as biting; or indirectly, by contaminating household surfaces, food or water. At a minimum, always take these precautions:

- Keep your home clean and free of debris. This will make it less attractive to pests.

SURVIVAL OF THE CLEANEST

- Drain, cover or treat stagnant water pools.
- Store food securely and correctly.
- Dispose of leftover food promptly and safely.
- Keep garbage in a securely covered bin.
- Block any potential entry points to your home.
- Follow the manufacturer's instructions for using pest control products and devices.
- Clean and disinfect any food preparation surfaces in an infested or treated area before use.

Guests

We shouldn't overlook or ignore the fact that our guests can bring harmful germs into our homes. Most of us cannot, and do not want to stop friends and family from visiting us at home. That said, we have to be aware that there is a contamination risk associated with receiving guests at home. To limit this risk, we need to understand what the specific threats are, learn how to mitigate them, and take the necessary steps to remove unavoidable contamination safely and effectively. We also need to accomplish all of this without offending our guests or making them feel uncomfortable, which makes things more complicated. Fortunately for us, common sense once again comes to the rescue. There are several steps we can take to safeguard our homes without alienating our friends and family:

- Be honest. Let your guests know upfront what your concerns and preferences are regarding health and household hygiene matters.

HYGIENE IN THE HOME

- Don't be over-zealous. Remember, you can always clean and disinfect, or throw away things after your guests have left.
- Make it easy for your guests to avoid contaminating your home:
  - Provide antibacterial soap, paper towels, disposable seat covers and disinfectant wipes in the bathroom.
  - If you frequently receive guests, consider installing touchless faucets and touchless paper towel dispensers in bathrooms and in the kitchen.
  - Place hand sanitizer dispensers in the bathroom, in the kitchen and in other strategic places around the house.
- Clean and disinfect bathrooms thoroughly after your guests have left.
- Remove and launder sheets and towels immediately after overnight guests have left.
- Vacuum carpets and upholstery. Pay special attention to areas where guests placed their luggage.
- Wash and disinfect floors.

PETS & WILD ANIMALS

Pets

Household pets such as dogs, cats, birds and reptiles can carry infectious germs and parasites that make people sick. The good news is that most pet-to-people diseases can be avoided if you follow a few common sense rules.

Preventing Infection

There are a number of precautions you can take to protect your family from the diseases transmitted by pets:

- Avoid touching your animal's urine or feces, or any surfaces contaminated by animal waste. Use a spade or a scoop to pick up dog waste from the lawn.
- Always wash your hands thoroughly immediately after picking up animal waste, cleaning a soiled carpet or cleaning a cat litter box. Teach children to do the same. Remember to clean under your fingernails.
- Don't kiss a pet on the mouth.
- Never share food with a pet or touch food that has been in contact with a pet's mouth.

PETS & WILD ANIMALS

- People with impaired or weakened immune systems, sick people, pregnant women and young children should never clean or handle cat litter boxes. Soiled cat litter can spread a very serious disease called toxoplasmosis. Toxoplasmosis can cause severe birth defects in an unborn child if the mother is infected during pregnancy.
- Do not keep reptiles as pets. They can spread life-threatening infections to humans.
- Keep your pets healthy:
  - Clean pet living areas at least once a week. Disinfect surfaces with a chlorine bleach solution or use a cleaning product that contains a disinfectant. Wash pet bedding in hot water and set the dryer at the highest temperature. I recommend using a detergent that contains bleach, or adding bleach to the water.
  - Food and water bowls should be washed daily. Use an antibacterial dish soap for extra protection. Each pet should have its own food and water bowls.
  - Cat litter boxes should be cleaned daily, the dirty litter placed in a plastic bag and discarded in the trash. Add baking soda to the litter to absorb odours.
  - Keep your pets under a veterinarian's care for regular vaccinations, deworming and dental cleaning. This not only keeps your pet healthy; it also reduces your risk of contracting diseases from your pet. If the cost of veterinary care is an issue, contact a local animal shelter or the SPCA for information about low-cost clinics.
  - Feed your pet a balanced diet and do not allow it to drink out of the toilet.

SURVIVAL OF THE CLEANEST

- ■ Keep your pets healthy (continued)
  - Control fleas and ticks on your pets and in your house. Fleas and ticks can make both you and your pets sick.
  - Don't feed raw meat to your pets. Do not allow your cats to hunt and eat mice. This is how they get the toxoplasmosis parasite. Keep your pets away from wild animals or stray pets.
  - Adopt pets from an animal shelter or buy them from a reputable pet store or breeder.
  - Have new pets examined right away by a veterinarian.
- ■ Protect children from pet-borne diseases:
  - Supervise small children while they play with pets. They are more likely to contract infections from pets because they crawl around on the floor with the animals, kiss them, put their fingers in the pets' mouths, and might then put their dirty fingers in their own mouths.
  - Small children are also more likely to be bitten or scratched by pets, since they treat pets as toys. Teach your children how to treat family pets and to avoid strange pets. It may be safest to wait to get a pet until children are past the toddler stage.
  - Don't let children handle reptiles and don't keep a reptile as a pet.
  - Keep children's sandboxes covered when not in use. A sandbox can quickly become a cat's litter box. Don't let small children play in uncovered sandboxes.
  - Any areas that may be contaminated with dog or cat feces should be off-limits to children, including at home and in parks, playgrounds or at the beach. Teach children not to eat dirt.

PETS & WILD ANIMALS

■ If you're planning to get a pet, consider adopting an older cat or dog, instead of getting a puppy or kitten. This way you can avoid the housebreaking stage and its problems. Older pets that have been well cared for are less likely to spread disease or become ill themselves. Be careful when taking in sick pets or stray animals; they pose a higher risk of infecting you or your children.

Pet Birds

Although illness caused by touching or owning birds is rare, birds can spread germs to people. The best protection against infection is to thoroughly wash your hands with hot water and soap immediately after handling birds, cages, food and water bowls.

Different species of birds can carry different pathogens. Baby chicks and ducklings often carry *Salmonella* bacteria, the cause of salmonellosis in people. Parakeets and parrots can carry the bacterium *Chlamydia psittaci*. This germ causes the disease psittacosis. Pigeon droppings can be contaminated with several germs that cause illness in people.

Some people are more at risk of being infected by birds. Older people, children younger than five years old, organ transplant patients, people with HIV/AIDS, and people being treated for cancer are more likely to contract diseases from birds. Children under five should not be allowed to touch baby chicks and ducklings. These birds can infect children with *Salmonella*.

Reptiles

I strongly advise against keeping reptiles as pets. Reptiles like snakes, lizards and turtles pose a high risk for salmonellosis and other serious infections. According to the US Centers for Disease Control and Prevention (CDC), pet reptiles and amphibians are responsible for about 93,000 *Salmonella* infections in the USA each year.

Young children have an increased risk of contracting *Salmonella* from pet reptiles and of developing serious, potentially fatal, complications from the infection. A study by the University of Michigan, published in *Clinical Infectious Diseases,* found that reptiles caught in the wild or bought at a pet store often carry *Salmonella* bacteria.

If, in spite of the dangers, you choose to keep a reptile as a pet, pay close attention to these precautions:

- Wash your hands thoroughly after handling a reptile, amphibian, its cage or food bowl. This becomes even more critical when there are children in the house.
- Ensure that children wash their hands after handling or feeding reptiles.
- Reptile pets should not be allowed to roam freely in the house and their enclosures should be kept clean.
- Reptiles should not be kept in homes with children under age five or in homes with people who have compromised immune systems.
- If you are expecting a child, remove the reptile or amphibian from the home before the child is born.

PETS & WILD ANIMALS

- Do not allow reptiles or amphibians in the kitchen or other food preparation areas.
- Do not wash reptiles, amphibians, their cages or their dishes in the kitchen sink. If the bathtub is used for that purpose, clean and disinfect it thoroughly with chlorine bleach.
- Teach children not to handle pet reptiles owned by their friends.

Wild Animals

Avoid contact with wild animals at all times. Keep your children and pets away from wild animals.

- Rodents can transmit hantavirus and plague.
- Ticks on animals can transmit tick paralysis, Rocky Mountain Spotted Fever and Lyme disease.
- Animals such as raccoons, squirrels, bats and coyotes can transmit rabies.

Precautions

There are a number of steps you can take to protect your family from contact with wild animals:

- Most wild animals come out at night and are afraid of people. If you see a wild animal during the day, you should avoid any contact with it and notify animal control authorities. The animal may have rabies.
- Keep food containers and garbage bins closed with tight-fitting lids at all times.

SURVIVAL OF THE CLEANEST

- Discard any excess pet food and keep food and water bowls inside the house.
- Discourage animals from entering or nesting in your house:
  - Keep doors and windows closed.
  - Eliminate any possible nesting sites and items that provide a water source.
  - Seal entrances on the inside and the outside of your home. A mouse can squeeze through an opening as small as a dime.
  - Female rats can have as many as 60 offspring in a year. Under ideal conditions, a single pair of Norway rats can produce 15,000 offspring in one year! One pair of mice can produce up to 8,000 offspring per year. You can keep rodent populations low by continually setting traps inside and outside your home.
  - Keep baits and traps out of reach of children and pets.
  - If your home is infested with rodents, contact animal control authorities.
  - Keep your home clean.
- If you find a dead animal:
  - Spray the animal with a disinfectant before moving it. This reduces the risk of exposure to deadly viruses.
  - Wear disposable gloves when moving the carcass and wash and disinfect your hands afterwards.

*****

PETS & WILD ANIMALS

Animal Bites and Scratches

Several million people are victims of animal bites each year in Canada and the United States. Approximately one percent of these bites result in hospitalization. Dog bites account for 80% to 85% of all reported incidents. Cats account for about ten percent of all reported bites, and other animals, including rodents, rabbits, horses, raccoons, mules, skunks, bats and monkeys make up the remaining five to ten percent.

The most common problem resulting from an animal bite is *wound infection*. Animal saliva contains a wide variety of bacteria and other germs. When an animal bites you, pathogens can enter the wound. Bacteria can grow inside the wound and cause infection. The consequences of infection range from pain and discomfort to potentially deadly complications.

Cat bites are more likely to become infected than dog bites. Because dogs have rounded teeth and strong jaws, their bites usually result in crush injuries. The canine teeth in a dog's mouth are sharp and can inflict lacerations. Cats have needle-like incisors and carnassial teeth, and typically cause puncture wounds. Cat teeth basically inject bacteria into the bite area, and the deep, narrow wounds are difficult to clean and disinfect.

Some of the bacteria typically found in animal bite wounds are *Pasteurella multocida*, *Staphylococcus aureus*, *Pseudomonas sp.* and *Streptococcus sp*. The cause of pasteurellosis, *P. multocida*, is often present in cat bite infections. Animal bite wounds also contain anaerobic germs. These microbes live and multiply in the absence of oxygen. A study published in 2003 found that as many as two-thirds of animal bite wounds contain anaerobes. They cause diseases like septic arthritis, meningitis and infections of the lymphatic system.

The most visible sign of infection from an animal bite is inflammation. The skin surrounding the wound is red and warm, and pus may drain from the wound. Nearby lymph glands may be swollen.

If the infection is left untreated, bacteria can enter the bloodstream and cause potentially fatal complications far away from the wound site, including meningitis, brain abscesses, pneumonia, lung abscesses and heart infections.

Other serious infectious diseases from animal bites include cat-scratch disease, tetanus and rabies. These diseases are discussed in more detail below.

Cat-scratch disease is caused by *Bartonella henselae* bacteria present in cat saliva. An estimated 40 percent of cats are infected with *B. henselae* at some point in their lives. However, cats do not show any symptoms of the disease, so it isn't possible to tell which cats are carriers.

You can become infected if a cat bites or scratches you. Symptoms can include swollen lymph nodes, fever, headache, fatigue, rash and loss of appetite. According to the US Centers for Disease Control and Prevention (CDC), approximately 22,000 cases are reported each year in the United States. The disease is not normally serious in healthy individuals, but symptoms may be severe in individuals with compromised immunity, such as people with HIV/AIDS or cancer.

Tetanus is caused by the toxin produced by *Clostridium tetani* bacteria. It affects the central nervous system and can be fatal. *Clostridium tetani* spores are found in soil and dust. The spores enter the body through a break in the skin, such as a cut or puncture wound. Animal bites and scratches can cause tetanus. The spores germinate inside the body and release active bacteria that produce the toxin. If left untreated, *one in three* people will die from tetanus. For babies and infants the prognosis is even bleaker: *two out of three* will die.

Tetanus symptoms include:

- Stiff jaw, neck and other muscles.
- Rigidity of chest, back and abdominal muscles.
- Back muscle spasms and arching of the back.
- Painful seizures.
- Fever and excessive sweating.
- Difficulty to swallow and drooling.
- Foot or hand spasms.
- Uncontrolled urination and defecation.

The most important weapon against tetanus is vaccination. Most people receive their first tetanus shot in childhood. Immunization provides protection for ten years. Booster shots are given to teenagers and adults.

Seek immediate medical attention for puncture-type injuries if your last immunization was more than ten years ago, or if you are unsure of your tetanus immunization status. If you thoroughly clean and disinfect wounds you can reduce the risk of developing tetanus.

Rabies is the deadliest disease that animals can transmit to people. Human rabies is rare in North America, but it is always fatal once symptoms appear. The World Health Organization (WHO) estimates that between 35,000 and 50,000 individuals worldwide die each year as a result of rabies.

After decades of vaccination, rabies in domestic pets has been virtually eliminated in the United States and Canada. However, it is still prevalent among wild animals. Dogs, as well as cats, should be immunized against rabies. This will protect them against rabies if they are attacked by a rabid animal. If your pet is not immunized, it could contract rabies and infect you and your family. You should also keep your pets under control to avoid contact with wild animals.

Symptoms of rabies in animals include abnormal behaviour, excessive salivation and paralysis. Symptoms of rabies in humans include abnormal behaviour, fever, anxiety, severe muscle spasms and an inability to swallow.

The good news is that rabies can almost always be prevented, even after exposure. Awareness and prompt preventive treatment are essential. If there is a risk of rabies, immune globulin and a course of vaccination are given to the bite victim to prevent the disease. Seek immediate medical help! Because rabies is caused by a virus, antibiotics are not effective.

People with a high risk of contracting rabies, for example veterinarians, animal handlers and laboratory workers, should receive pre-exposure vaccination.

PETS & WILD ANIMALS

Precautions

■ Prevent bites and scratches:
- Supervise small children and teach them how to behave appropriately around pets and other animals.
- Avoid 'rough play,' especially with cats.
- Avoid any animals that are unusually aggressive or behaving strangely (for example a raccoon that is active during the daytime). Immediately contact your local animal control authorities; the animal may be infected with the rabies virus.
- Don't take in wild animals as pets.
- Don't leave food, garbage or pet food that might attract wild animals outside the home or campsite.
- Never try to break up fights between animals.
- Avoid unknown cats and dogs.
- Animals should not be trained to fight.

■ Domestic pets should be vaccinated against rabies; consult a veterinarian for advice about the frequency of booster vaccinations for the area in which you live.

■ People who are traveling to countries where rabies is endemic should consider vaccination.

■ If you are bitten or scratched by an animal:
- Wash animal bites and scratches with hot, running water and antibacterial soap.
- Apply antibacterial medication and cover the wound.
- If you develop symptoms of an infection, contact your doctor as soon as possible.

Petting Zoos and Farm Animals

Petting zoo animals and farm animals are carriers of many different germs, including a strain of *E. coli* bacteria that can cause a life-threatening kidney disease, called Haemolytic Uremic Syndrome, or HUS. This strain of *E. coli* can survive for as long as 30 days in soil and on animals. People can become infected if they touch farm animals or petting zoo animals. Young children visiting petting zoos are particularly at risk; their immune systems are less capable of fighting infection.

Precautions

The obvious way to prevent animal-borne diseases is to avoid farm animals and to keep your kids away from petting zoos. That would be my first choice. I do, however, realize that many people enjoy being around farm animals, or live in a rural setting, and that most parents do not want to deny their small children the experience of interacting with animals in the petting zoo. You should not ignore the risks, though. Always take the necessary precautions and exercise extreme caution around petting zoos and farm animals.

At a minimum, always take the following precautions:

- Carry sufficient hand sanitizer or antibacterial wipes for everybody in your group. Use liberally after touching any animals.
- Never leave young children unsupervised with petting zoo or farm animals. Make sure their mouths

and faces do not come into contact with animals, and that they don't touch their mouths, eyes or noses.
- Don't eat or drink while handling or touching animals. It goes without saying that children should not be allowed to eat or drink while they are in contact with animals.
- Always, always, *always* wash and/or sanitize your hands after being in contact with animals. Never eat, drink, touch your face or handle food before washing and/or sanitizing your hands. Children should be supervised and assisted to ensure that their hands are thoroughly disinfected.
- Before visiting a petting zoo, contact local authorities to find out if there have been any outbreaks of *E. coli* or other health-related issues at the facility you plan to visit.

INSECTS

Insects are not just annoying; many carry and spread the germs that cause infectious diseases such as West Nile disease, Lyme disease and malaria. While ticks and mosquitoes pose the biggest danger in North America, other insects like flies also carry infectious germs.

Worldwide, an estimated one person in every six is infected with an insect-borne disease. The Encyclopædia Britannica lists insects as carriers of the pathogens that cause most major human fevers.

Insects can spread many different types of micro-organisms, including bacteria, viruses and protozoa that cause infectious diseases. The micro-organisms are the pathogens and the insects involved are known as vectors.

Insects act as vectors (transmitters of disease) in two ways:

- **Mechanical transmission of external germs** – Insects like cockroaches and houseflies carry germs on their feet. For example, flies can pick up traces of feces and infect people with debilitating and deadly illnesses such as typhoid, dysentery and cholera when they land on our food or drinks. Flies can also spread trachoma, the primary cause of blindness in the developing world. Cockroaches thrive in filth and mechanically transmit disease to humans.

- **Mechanical transmission of internal pathogens** – When insects harbour viruses, bacteria or parasites inside their bodies, they can infect us through a bite or other means. For example, mosquitoes can transmit West Nile virus and malaria, the world's second deadliest infectious disease (tuberculosis is the number one killer). Tick bites can cause Lyme disease, tick paralysis, Colorado tick fever, tularemia and other serious illnesses.

Disease-carrying Insects

Flies

The housefly is found virtually everywhere on the globe. It is a major health hazard, especially in areas where sanitation is poor. They carry germs of several deadly diseases and cause millions of deaths every year.

Flies feed by first releasing saliva and digestive juices over food and then sponging up the resulting solution. It goes without saying that flies contaminate large amounts of food because of the way they eat.

Flies also contaminate food by rubbing their legs together. They do this to clean themselves. Dirt and harmful germs removed from their legs by this process can end up in our food and drinks and infect us. Houseflies leave germs everywhere they land. Some of the diseases spread by the housefly are food poisoning, typhoid, tuberculosis and dysentery. These diseases can cause death if they are left untreated.

Flies usually live and breed in garbage and sewage. The female lays about 100 eggs at a time and as many as 750 during her lifetime. The eggs hatch into larvae in 12 to 30 hours. Within a few days, the pupae become adults and the cycle begins again. Most houseflies have a lifespan of 15 to 25 days. Cold weather usually kills off the adults, but larvae and pupae are able to survive the winter. If all the eggs laid by a housefly were to mature, one fly could have more than 300,000 grandchildren. Fortunately, only a small percentage of eggs survive, but still enough to pose a serious threat to our health.

Protecting Against Flies

Here are some guidelines for controlling flies:

- Keep your home clean.
- Store food or anything that attracts insects in covered food storage containers.
- If you have dogs, pick up their waste daily and discard it safely.
- Clean cat litter boxes and other pet cages daily.
- In order to stop breeding, start controlling houseflies in early spring.
- Keep dustbins clean and regularly treat them with insecticide. Ensure that lids fit tightly.
- Ensure that all food, and eating and cooking utensils are protected from houseflies.

INSECTS

- Keep the house entirely free from flies, particularly where there are babies and people with weakened immune systems.
- Keep garden waste and compost heaps far away from the house.

Mosquitoes

According to the World Health Organization (WHO), of all disease-transmitting insects, the mosquito is the greatest menace, spreading malaria, dengue and yellow fever. Together, these diseases are responsible for several million deaths and hundreds of millions of cases of illness every year. At least 40 percent of the earth's population is at risk for malaria, and about 40 percent for dengue fever. In many places, people can contract both. Mosquitoes transmit diseases such as:

- West Nile disease
- Malaria
- Dengue and dengue haemorrhagic fever
- Encephalitis
- Rift Valley fever
- Filariasis
- Yellow fever

Protecting Against Mosquitoes

When entering a region where any of the above diseases are endemic, you should take the following precautions:

SURVIVAL OF THE CLEANEST

- Avoid bites by wearing long-sleeved clothing and long trousers.
- Use an effective insect repellent. Products that contain the chemical DEET as active ingredient provide the best protection. Mosquitoes are attracted to humans by the body's moisture, warmth, odour and the release of carbon dioxide. Repellents work by blocking receptors on mosquito antennae that sense these attractants. To be effective, repellent has to be applied to all exposed skin. Mosquitoes can readily find and bite untreated areas.
- Most insects can bite through thin clothing, so spray repellent on them.
- To control mosquitoes indoors, spray DEET repellent or an insecticide, burn pyrethroid coils or heat insecticide impregnated tablets.
- Always use a mosquito net impregnated with insecticide when sleeping outside or in an unscreened room. Packable, lightweight nets are available from outdoor equipment stores.
- Eliminate mosquito breeding sites: cover water tanks and washtubs, eliminate open containers that collect water and don't let water stand in potted plants. Mosquitoes can breed in any puddle standing four days or more.
- Certain fragrances attract insects, so avoid scented soaps and hygiene products.
- Products like garlic, vitamin B and ultrasound devices do not prevent mosquito bites.

INSECTS

Ticks

With the exception of mosquitoes, ticks can transmit more diseases to humans than any other insect. A single tick can harbour as many as three different infectious germs and transmit all of them in one bite. Ticks can carry Lyme disease, the most common vector-borne illness in North America and Europe.

There are more than 850 tick species worldwide and 30 major tick-borne diseases. There are over 80 species of ticks in North America that collectively can cause several serious diseases. These diseases include:

- Lyme Disease
- Ehrlichiosis
- Babesiosis
- Tick Paralysis
- Tick-borne Relapsing Fever
- Tularemia
- Rocky Mountain Spotted Fever
- Colorado Tick Fever

Most of these diseases have symptoms similar to the flu, such as fever, chills, headache, muscle ache, vomiting and fatigue.

In North America, the tick-borne disease that causes most concern is Lyme Disease, an infectious disease that is spread by deer ticks found in most wooded areas in northeast and northcentral North America. Infection is caused by a bacterium that is transmitted to humans by tick bites. Early symptoms include an expanding red rash at the site of the bite, severe headache, muscle and joint aches, and high fever.

The risk of being bitten by an infected tick is greatest in summer. This is also the time of year when most people are active outdoors. You should be aware of the symptoms of tick-borne diseases and take preventive measures to reduce the danger of infection from ticks.

Protecting Against Tick Bites

Always take the following precautions when spending time in tick-infested areas:

- Avoid tick habitats if possible.
- Make a habit of thoroughly checking yourself and others for ticks after outdoor activities. Spot-check yourself and others frequently for ticks on clothes; if you find one, there may be others.
- Wear light-coloured clothing with a tight weave to spot ticks more easily and prevent contact with the skin.
- Always wear closed shoes.
- Wear clothes that minimize exposed skin, especially when in the woods. Wear long pants tucked into socks, long-sleeved shirts tucked into pants.
- Apply tick repellent to your clothes and skin. Products that contain DEET or Permethrin are known to offer effective protection.
- Carefully read the manufacturer's directions and cautions before using a tick repellent.
- Keep your pets healthy and free of ticks.

INSECTS

- Keep long hair pulled back in the garden or in the outdoors.
- When gardening, pruning shrubs, or working with soil and vegetation, wear light-coloured gloves, and spot-check them for ticks frequently.
- Avoid sitting directly on the ground and stay on cleared, well-worn trails whenever possible.
- Remove clothes after leaving tick-infested areas and, if possible, wash and dry them to eliminate any unseen ticks.
- Conduct a full-body check of yourself, your children and any outdoor pets from head to toe for ticks each night before going to bed. Be sure to check the scalp, behind the head and neck, in the ears, the groin area and behind joints.
- If you find a tick, it should be removed with tweezers. Pull firmly and steadily on the tick until it lets go, then swab the bite site with alcohol or other disinfectant.
- Keep the tick in a bottle labeled with the person's name, location of bite site and the date.
- Don't use petroleum jelly or a lit match to kill and remove a tick.
- Monitor the tick bite site and seek medical attention if you notice a rash or any other symptoms of a tick-borne illness.

*****

Fleas

Fleas can be hosts for tapeworms, encephalitis, typhoid, tularemia and plague. Also known as Black Death, plague wiped out a third of the European population during the Middle Ages in just six years, and continues to kill people to this day.

Protecting Against Fleas

- Keep your home free of fleas. Vacuum all carpets regularly and use an appropriate insecticide. Always follow the directions for use.
- Call a professional pest control service if you have a major infestation of fleas.
- Keep your pets free of fleas. Bathe them regularly and consult your vet or pet clinic about suitable flea control products.
- Keep your property free of rats and other rodents. Rat fleas can spread plague from rats to humans.
- If you can't control your environment, for example when traveling, use insect repellent to protect yourself and use an insecticide to rid your immediate surroundings of fleas.
- Avoid stray dogs or cats. It goes without saying that rats and mice should be avoided at all times.
- Flea bites should be disinfected with an effective disinfectant, like alcohol or iodine. An over-the-counter cortisone or antihistamine product can be applied to relieve itching. Never scratch flea bites!

- If you develop any symptoms following a flea bite, such as rash, fever, headache or respiratory problems, seek immediate medical attention.

Other Insects

- Tsetse flies cause sleeping sickness.
- Blackflies carry river blindness and filariasis.
- Lice and mites can transmit typhus.
- Sandflies carry Leishmaniasis.
- Assassin or kissing bugs cause Chagas disease.

General Precautions

- Travelers should get the latest information on risks. Data is available from public health departments and government Internet sites. Take preventive treatment appropriate for the area/s you plan to visit.
- If you feel sick, seek medical attention. Insect-borne diseases can mimic other illnesses. Give your doctor a complete history.
- Clothing is the safest insect repellent. Make sure that your neck, ankles and wrists are protected. Choose fabrics with a tight weave and wear light-coloured clothing, which is less attractive to biting insects than dark clothing.
- Stay away from perfumed lotions, as certain smells can attract even more insects.
- Check clothes regularly for insects.

SURVIVAL OF THE CLEANEST

- Protective netting around sleeping and eating areas is an effective way to keep insects at bay.
- When visiting an area with a large insect population, always use insect repellent.
- Whenever you find yourself in mosquito, sand fly or tick territory, using chemical insect repellents become necessary. The most effective repellents contain the chemicals DEET, Permethrin, Indalone, Rutgers 612 or DMP. The active ingredient R-326 protects against biting flies.
- When you need to use both sunscreen and an insect repellent, apply the sunscreen first, then wait 30 minutes before applying the insect repellent.
- To avoid toxicity from insect repellents:
  - Apply repellent sparingly and only to exposed skin or clothing.
  - Keep repellent out of your eyes.
  - Avoid using high concentration products on the skin, particularly with children.
  - Never inhale or ingest repellents.
  - Wear long-sleeved clothing and apply the repellent to fabric rather than to your skin.
  - Wash off repellent when you are no longer at risk of being bitten by an insect. Repellent should never be used on children's hands because they are likely to rub their eyes or touch their mouths. Children two years old and younger should not have repellent applied to their skin more than once in a 24-hour period.

INSECTS

The DEET Debate

Insect repellents come in many forms: liquid, lotion, stick, gel, aerosol spray and wristbands. The most effective products are those that contain some concentration of the chemical N,N-diethyl-m-toluamide, commonly known as DEET. DEET offers protection against mosquitoes, ticks and other insects. Products containing 25 percent DEET provide protection for up to six hours.

Some people are concerned about exposing themselves or their children to DEET. However, DEET has been around for decades and has an excellent safety record. If used correctly, its effectiveness for preventing mosquito- or tick-borne illnesses far outweigh the small risk of toxicity.

DEET was developed by the US Department of Agriculture in 1946 and has been registered with the Environmental Protection Agency as an approved active ingredient since 1957. People have used it without demonstrable harm for decades. In rare instances, DEET has been responsible for skin irritation or inflammation when it was misused.

If you don't want to, or cannot use a product that contains DEET, because of a skin irritation or wound, other products offer limited protection. These repellents use plant-based oils such as oil of geranium, cedar, lemon grass, soy or citronella to repel insects. Plant-based repellents are effective for a much shorter period of time compared to DEET-based repellents.

Using DEET Safely

To avoid any possible adverse effects, follow these guidelines:

- Always follow directions. Before applying DEET to your skin, make sure that you've read the safety instructions on the container.
- Choose a product with the right amount of DEET. The higher the DEET concentration, the longer the protection lasts. Products containing 30 percent DEET or more are not recommended for children.
- Use the lowest effective concentration of DEET. A light repellent may be adequate for spending an hour or two in the backyard. Hiking in the woods or near surface water will require a repellent with a higher DEET concentration.
- Consider what types of biting insects are found in the area and how likely those insects are to carry disease.
- Apply repellent in moderation. While it is important to thoroughly cover all exposed skin, don't overdo it. Children under age two should have no more than one application of repellent a day.
- Never apply repellent to cut, scraped, sunburned or otherwise damaged skin.
- Don't use it on infants less than two months of age. Instead, cover your infant's stroller or playpen with mosquito netting when outside.
- Avoid getting insect repellent on the face and hands. It can easily get into the eyes from the hands, causing severe discomfort.

INSECTS

- Don't spray in a closed room. Apply insect repellent outdoors or in a well-ventilated room.
- Don't let children apply their own insect repellent. Children are likely to go overboard, using far more than necessary and increasing the risk that they'll get repellent in their eyes or mouths.
- Avoid using combination sunscreen/insect repellent products. Sunscreen should be applied freely and repeatedly; insect repellent should be applied sparingly. You need one product to ward off insect bites, and another to prevent sunburn.
- Wash off repellent when you're safely away from insects.
- DEET can damage plastics, synthetic fabrics, leather, and painted or varnished materials; avoid contact with eyeglasses, watch straps, walls and furniture. DEET doesn't harm nylon or natural fibers, such as cotton and wool.

DEET is the most effective mosquito and tick repellent currently available. It is safe as long as you choose the appropriate concentration and use it with common sense. If you accidentally inhale or swallow DEET, or have an adverse skin reaction, follow first-aid instructions for poisoning and seek medical attention.

DEET Alternatives

The US Centers for Disease Control and Prevention (CDC) has always recommended the chemical DEET as the most effective defence against mosquitoes. In 2005, the agency added two ingredients, *picaridin* and *oil of lemon eucalyptus,* as alternative repellents that offer effective protection against mosquitoes. Both products have been available elsewhere in the world, including Europe and Australia, since the 1980s. Repellents with DEET remain first on the CDC's recommendation list. In North America, DEET has always been the chemical of choice for health officials trying to control the spread of West Nile virus. The use of alternative repellents to prevent West Nile disease has never been recommended by the CDC and other public health authorities.

Some people dislike DEET's odour and others find it unpleasant on the skin. DEET repellents can damage plastic and synthetic fabrics. There has always been controversy around DEET's safety, although the US Environmental Protection Agency insists that it won't cause any harm to people if used properly.

Picaridin repellents tend to feel more pleasant on the skin and do not have the strong chemical odour that DEET repellents have. Oil of lemon eucalyptus is a natural ingredient, which appeals to people who dislike applying chemicals to their skin. The CDC recently reported that picaridin is 'often comparable with DEET products of similar concentration' and that oil of lemon eucalyptus provides protection time 'similar to low-concentration DEET products.'

Whether you choose a DEET-based or an alternative repellent, always take additional personal protection measures, such as wearing long-sleeved clothing while outside and emptying containers of water that could be breeding grounds for mosquitoes.

Insects and HIV

Insects do not transmit HIV. Extensive research done by medical scientists and entomologists failed to find any evidence that mosquitoes, or any other insects for that matter, transmit the virus. Studies done by the CDC and international research organizations, in parts of the world where both AIDS and mosquitoes are prevalent, have produced no evidence of HIV outbreaks caused by mosquitoes or other insects.

There are many factors that make it impossible for mosquitoes to infect people with HIV. A mosquito's mouth has two openings. It draws blood in through one passage and delivers saliva through the other. This means it cannot re-inject blood when it bites the next person. Furthermore, any viruses ingested by the mosquito are destroyed when its digestive system breaks down the blood. HIV also does not infiltrate the mosquito's salivary glands, as in the case of malaria and yellow fever.

To become infected with HIV, a person must be exposed to a large number of infectious particles. When a mosquito flies directly from one person to another, the amount of blood on its mouth is too small to result in infection with HIV. Even swatting a mosquito filled with HIV-positive blood over an open wound would not cause HIV infection.

The virus lives for only a short time outside the human body and does not reproduce in insects. This means that insects do not become infected and cannot transmit HIV to the next person they bite.

GARDENING

Gardening is a wonderful, relaxing and rewarding pastime that should certainly not be avoided. However, working in the garden comes with a number of risks for infection and becoming sick. Fortunately, by taking a few simple precautions, you can continue to enjoy gardening without jeopardizing your health.

Germs lurk everywhere in the typical suburban garden. Bacteria, viruses, fungi and parasites are present in soil and water in immense numbers: a handful of soil contains billions of micro-organisms. Potentially deadly bacteria like *E. coli 0157:H7, Salmonella, Campylobacter*, and the bacteria that cause botulism and tetanus are commonly found in soil. Parasites like *Cryptosporidium* and *Giardia*, and a variety of fungi and viruses live in the soil, water and on plants.

Many pathogens can survive in the environment for extended periods. Some, for example botulism bacteria, develop a spore or cyst that has the ability to survive when it is excreted or shed by their original host. Others, like *E. coli 0157:H7* and *Salmonella* bacteria can survive in frozen soil for many months, as long as ten months in the case of *E. coli 0157:H7*. Our cold winter weather offers no protection against these germs.

GARDENING

Tetanus and botulism, potentially the two most deadly diseases a gardener can contract, are discussed in more detail below.

Tetanus

Tetanus, also known as lockjaw, is a bacterial disease that affects the nervous system. It is contracted through a cut or wound that becomes contaminated with tetanus bacteria. The bacteria can get in through even a tiny pinprick or scratch, but deep puncture wounds or cuts like those made by rusty nails or knives are especially susceptible to infection with tetanus. Tetanus bacteria are present worldwide and are commonly found in soil, dust and manure. Infection with tetanus causes severe muscle spasms, leading to 'locking' of the jaw so that the patient cannot open his or her mouth or swallow, and may even lead to death by suffocation. Thanks to immunization, tetanus is now quite rare, but without immunization there is still a real chance of contracting the disease. It is important for adults to keep their tetanus vaccinations up to date. Check with your doctor when you last had a tetanus vaccination.

Botulism

Botulism is a paralytic illness caused by a deadly toxin produced by *Clostridium botulinum* bacteria. Botulism bacteria are found in soil and water, in fish, and on marine animals.

Botulism toxin is one of the deadliest poisons in the world. One teaspoon of pure botulism poison can kill thousands of people. A mere taste of contaminated food can make you very, very sick.

There are three primary kinds of botulism. Foodborne botulism is caused by eating foods that contain the botulism toxin. Wound botulism is caused by toxin produced from a wound infected with *Clostridium botulinum*. Infant botulism is caused by ingesting the spores of the botulism bacteria, which then grow in the intestines and release toxin. All forms of botulism can be fatal and should be considered medical emergencies.

The bacteria themselves are completely harmless, until they find the right growing conditions for producing their poison. They form a protective coating and become spores. This allows the germs to survive until they find suitable conditions in which they can grow and start producing botulism toxin.

Symptoms of botulism poisoning include double vision, drooping eyelids, slurred speech, dry mouth, difficulty swallowing and muscle weakness.

Safe Gardening Practices

By following the guidelines in this chapter, gardeners can greatly reduce their exposure to harmful germs, as well as to other potentially harmful materials such as pesticides that might be in the soil.

Working in the Garden

- Wear sturdy gardening gloves to protect your hands from cuts and scratches.

GARDENING

- Avoid eating or drinking while working in the yard or garden. Contaminated soil and dust might get on your food and you could accidentally swallow it.
- Don't touch your eyes, nose or mouth while working in the garden.
- Dampen soil with water before you garden to limit the amount of dust you inhale.
- Avoid working in the yard on windy days, when dust can be stirred up and increase your exposure.
- Wear a protective face mask and goggles if you spend time in dusty areas.
- Wash your hands after gardening and before eating or handling food.
- Wash work clothes to remove dust and dirt.
- Take off your shoes at the door to avoid tracking soil into your home.
- Hydrogen peroxide is an environmentally safe alternative to bleach for sterilizing greenhouse and gardening equipment. Peroxide also reduces diseases on cuttings and seedlings. Mix one part three percent strength peroxide and eight parts of water.
- Isopropyl (rubbing) alcohol can be used to clean and disinfect work surfaces, tools and equipment used for gardening.
- Rusty garden tools can cause serious injuries that can lead to tetanus and other infections. Keep tools clean by scrubbing them with soap and water. Hand dry them or let them air dry, and store them in a dry place. Do not leave garden tools exposed to rain. Use

specifically formulated solvents, available from most hardware stores, to remove rust from garden tools. As an alternative, apply cola pop or vinegar with aluminum foil or use fine sandpaper to clean bare metal parts. Apply a light coat of vegetable oil to the metal parts of garden tools to prevent rust.

Preparing Fruits and Vegetables

Washing the soil from your homegrown fruit and vegetables is one of the most effective ways of reducing your exposure to germs, and other contaminants like pesticides and arsenic.

- Clean your hands, cutting boards and kitchen tools with hot, soapy water and rinse well before and after handling fruit and vegetables.
- Soak garden produce in clean, cold water and rinse thoroughly until the water runs clear. Commercial vegetable cleaning products are available to help free soil residues from produce. These products work well with leafy vegetables. Vinegar or a hydrogen peroxide solution can also be used for cleaning produce. To make a peroxide cleaning solution, add one part three percent strength hydrogen peroxide to eight parts of water. Use vinegar undiluted. Rinse the produce with clean water before eating or cooking.
- Scrub firm fruits and root crops with a cleaning brush to remove dust and dirt before peeling or eating.
- Peel root crops like carrots, potatoes, radishes and turnips before cooking or eating them.

GARDENING

- Wash berry fruits like strawberries and blackberries, and remove the tops of the berries where the stem and leaves are attached.

Safe Composting Practices

Compost can do wonders for your garden. A well-managed compost heap safely produces inexpensive and environmentally friendly compost; a badly managed compost heap can quickly turn into a health and sanitation nightmare.

A compost heap consists of decomposing organic matter. The resulting high temperatures and moist conditions provide the ideal environment for bacteria and fungi. Some of these microbes are necessary for the decomposition processes; others can cause dangerous infectious diseases.

Some compost heaps also contain animal manures. These are particularly dangerous since *E. coli, Salmonella, Campylobacter* and *Listeria* infections can be spread via animal feces. Tetanus bacteria are also found in manure.

Compost heaps also attract rats, mice, cockroaches, flies and other insects. These pests will soon infiltrate your house if you don't take proper care. Cockroaches and flies carry the germs that cause dysentery, gastroenteritis and typhoid.

Fortunately, safe composting is easily achievable if you follow the composting guidelines below:

- Place your compost heap or bin in an enclosed area, as far away from the house as possible.

SURVIVAL OF THE CLEANEST

- Keep the heap covered with a tarpaulin.
- Place several fly traps near the compost heap.
- Do not add meat, seafood or dairy waste to your compost heap. They take longer to break down and are more likely to attract rats and flies than plant material.
- Always wash your hands thoroughly after working with compost.
- Do not eat or drink while handling compost.
- Keep children and pets away from compost heaps. They may contract diseases and spread the germs inside the house.
- Place an open container with citronella oil next to the compost heap to keep flies away. If the flies become more tenacious, light a few citronella candles to chase them away.
- Chopping or shredding the organic material greatly reduces volume and decreases decomposing time.
- Do not add cat or dog waste to your compost bin or heap; it may contain parasites that can contaminate the compost.
- Do not add diseased plants to the compost heap. These harmful microbes may survive the composting process and infect healthy plants when the compost is used in the garden.
- Avoid contaminating compost with pesticides. The chemicals in the pesticides can affect the microbes in the compost heaps and slow down the natural composting process.

GARDENING

- Compost bins are safer than compost heaps because their enclosure keeps animals out. They also look tidier.
- To make bins animal proof consider the following:
  - Line the compost bins with wire mesh.
  - Add a secure or airtight lid.
  - Make ventilation holes no bigger than a quarter inch.
- It is preferable to construct compost systems from materials such as plastic, which can withstand harsh weather conditions.

Stagnant Water

If you live in an area where there is heavy rain and inadequate drainage, stagnant pools of water are going to be a problem before too long.

Pools of water are ideal territory for insects to lay their eggs in and for germs to proliferate. Mosquitoes, which can spread West Nile virus and other diseases, thrive in still-standing puddles of water. A dangerous strain of the *E. coli* bacteria also prefers wet environments. These bacteria can cause a deadly form of gastroenteritis. Other diseases that can be spread by means of still-standing water include typhoid fever, dysentery and cholera. The water features found in many gardens can also become breeding grounds for germs and insects if they are neglected. Water features should either be properly maintained or drained.

To stop insects and germs from getting a foothold in your garden, water sources should be treated, covered

SURVIVAL OF THE CLEANEST

up or drained. Take the following precautions if you have standing water on your property:

- If possible, drain pools of stagnant water and take steps to prevent them from filling up again.
- If draining is not an option, cover the water with a tarpaulin to keep insects and animals out, and to prevent children from coming into contact with it.
- If mosquitoes are a problem, mosquito larval oil can be poured onto the surface of stagnant water to kill off the pupae.
- Adding a cup of chlorine bleach to small pools of stagnant water should kill most germs.

LITTER

Litter is more than an unsightly blemish on the landscape. It also provides the perfect environment for germs to proliferate. In addition to its environmental impact, litter can directly threaten our health.

Litter can be defined as carelessly discarded garbage. It consists of fast food wrappers, paper, cigarette butts, plastic bottles, soda cans, coffee cups, glass bottles, plastic bags, candy wrappers and various other items we see next to roads, piled up against fences, on hiking trails, and on city sidewalks. We also find litter in our parks and on our beaches.

Sources seem to increase faster than people can be educated not to litter. Fast food packaging, the never-ending stream of junk mail, disposable consumer goods and elaborate packaging all contribute to the growing pile of garbage all around us. People's lifestyles have also changed: they are busier, engage in more snacking and increasingly rely on fast foods. This means more potential for litter in more places, more often.

Litter can be divided into four categories: *durable, offensive, unhygienic* and *dangerous*. Plastic bags, plastic bottles and fast food packaging are examples of durable litter. Cigarette butts and used condoms are the most common sources of offensive litter. Unhygienic litter sources include dog droppings and food waste. Syringes and broken bottles are examples of dangerous litter.

Litter and Germs

Litter is a breeding ground for disease. Because litter is exposed to the elements, it may start to decompose. In addition to causing a foul odour, decomposing litter provides a germ-friendly environment. Bacteria and other germs can multiply very rapidly in the right conditions. Flies, rats, mice, cockroaches and other scavenger animals are attracted to areas with lots of litter. They find their food among the trash, pick up germs and become carriers of infectious diseases.

Dangerous litter such as syringes and broken glass can infect us with deadly diseases, including hepatitis, HIV/AIDS and tetanus. Dog waste harbours a wide range of harmful bacteria and parasites. Food waste can spread *E. coli*, *Salmonella* and other diseases. Litter can end up in rivers, lakes and streams, and contaminate our drinking water with viruses, bacteria and parasites.

Stopping Litter

Although we cannot control other people's behaviour, there are several things we can do to reduce litter and the associated risk of germ contamination:

- Lead by example: Always properly dispose of your own garbage.

LITTER

- Recycle everything that can be recycled and put all other garbage in the proper containers.
- If a family member or friend throws something on the ground, ask them politely to place the item in a trash receptacle instead.
- If you see a piece of litter, pick it up and throw it away. But remember, never touch anything that may be sharp or hazardous.
- Join a group that cleans up local areas.
- Petition local authorities to place more trash bins where needed.
- Report illegal dumping to authorities.
- Petition political representatives to introduce stiffer penalties for littering, and to ensure consistent enforcement in your community.
- Educate your children about the health risks and environmental impact of littering.
- Always wear protective gloves when picking up litter, and wash and sanitize your hands thoroughly afterwards.

GERM ETIQUETTE

While the main focus of this book is on protecting ourselves and our families from infectious disease, it is also important to understand what we can do to prevent the spread of germs to other people. In addition to this being the right thing to do, we indirectly protect ourselves by being considerate to other people, because we help break the chain of infection. What doesn't go around, doesn't come around.

Practising germ etiquette is simple. The things we learned as children really work. They include covering your nose and mouth when you sneeze, cough, or blow your nose; using a tissue when possible; washing your hands frequently and thoroughly; and staying home when you are sick.

You can make a difference by practising these good health manners whenever you are ill:

- You have a responsibility to avoid infecting others.
- Let other people in the household or at work know when you are sick.
- Always cover your nose and mouth with a tissue when sneezing, coughing or blowing your nose. Safely dispose of used tissues as soon as possible.

GERM ETIQUETTE

- Always wash your hands after sneezing, blowing your nose or coughing, or after touching used tissues. Wash your hands more often if you are sick.
- Use warm water and soap or alcohol-based hand sanitizers to clean your hands.
- Stay at home if you have a cold or flu, or any other infectious disease.
- Clinic and hospital staff may ask you to wear a face mask in waiting areas and exam rooms if you have a fever, cough or other symptoms. Cooperate with them and follow their instructions to help stop the spread of germs.
- Don't share food, utensils or beverage containers with others. The same rule applies to things like cigarettes, towels, lipstick, toys, or anything else that might be contaminated with respiratory germs.
- Use your own pen to fill out forms, sign credit card receipts, etc.
- Maintain a safe distance from other family members when you are ill. Don't hug or kiss them or shake hands.
- Clean and disinfect surfaces or objects you may have contaminated with your flu viruses or other germs.
- Don't prepare meals for others or handle food if you are sick.
- Teach your children the basics of germ etiquette. Set a good example.
- Don't handle food items at the grocery store more than is necessary.

SURVIVAL OF THE CLEANEST

- We are all links in the chain of infection, some more so than others. People who frequently come into contact with lots of other people; for example, supermarket checkout staff and air hostesses, have a higher risk of contracting and passing on infectious diseases. Others, who work in high-risk occupations like healthcare and food service, have a higher risk due to the nature of their work. These people can (and should) play a very important role in breaking the chain of infection by practising preventive hygiene.

- Insist on germ etiquette and considerate behaviour from others. We don't think twice about asking someone to wear a seat belt in the car or to refrain from smoking in the house. Why is it then that we still hesitate to ask other people if they have washed their hands? There is no good reason why we should not be able to raise issues that concern our health, or request others to respect our right to a disease-free environment. Some people may still be offended, but that, too, will change as germ etiquette becomes part of our social fabric.

NEW TECHNOLOGY TO THE RESCUE?

During the First World War, scientists in Germany discovered that antimicrobial treatments for uniforms worn by soldiers engaged in trench warfare, lowered the incidence of secondary wound infections. However, it wasn't until after the introduction of Microban® that antimicrobial plastics and other antimicrobial materials started entering the mainstream of consumer products. The last few years have seen an explosion of new antimicrobial products onto the market, including toys, athletic and outdoor wear, plastic kitchen utensils, pens, food service products, medical products, building materials and many more.

Antimicrobial products are here to stay. As long as there are germs, there will no doubt be a demand for products that make the world a cleaner and safer place.

Naturally, not everybody is enthusiastic about antimicrobial materials. Some worry about the growth of antibacterial resistant germs; others are concerned about the toxicity of triclosan and other antimicrobials; and some feel that antimicrobial products create a false sense of security, leading people to neglect basic hygiene.

Regular and correct hand washing is, and will remain, the best way to prevent infectious disease. Also, an inexpensive chlorine bleach solution will always be one of the most effective ways to disinfect kitchen utensils and surfaces, even when compared to the new antimicrobial materials.

Antimicrobial Plastic

Antimicrobial plastics are increasingly used in consumer products such as cutting boards, toothbrushes, mattress covers and children's toys. These plastics are composed of polymers mixed with special disinfectants. The plastic releases the disinfectant gradually, killing bacteria, mold, algae, mildew and other fungi that come into contact with its surface. When the disinfectant runs out, the plastic permanently loses its germ-killing ability.

Microban® is the best known antimicrobial plastic. It is manufactured using a special process that bonds triclosan to plastic polymers. Microban® is used in specialty products such as surgical drapes, orthopedic cast liners and hospital mattress covers. It is also used in a wide range of industrial, institutional, and consumer products. Other examples of the large number and variety of products that incorporate Microban® include dental instrument trays, socks, bedding, food-service wipes and industrial drains. The list of products continues to grow, thanks to the demand by companies seeking to infuse antimicrobial properties into their products, and the growing public awareness of the dangers of infectious germs and disease.

NEW TECHNOLOGY TO THE RESCUE?

Because triclosan works by penetrating cell walls, it is difficult for microbes to build up an immunity to it. This can make Microban® an important tool in the fight against drug-resistant bacteria. It is known to inhibit the growth of methicillin-resistant *Staphylococcus aureus* (MRSA) and four other strains of *Staphylococcus aureus*. Microban® is also effective against several strains of *Staphylococcus epidermis*, as well as two strains of *Enterococcus faecalis*.

Antimicrobial materials like Microban® will be used increasingly in the fight against hospital-acquired infections. Washrooms, drains and flooring in decontamination rooms, countertops in food preparation areas, food service utensils, steps, handrails, toilet seats, trash receptacles, shower cubicles and tiles can all be manufactured or coated with materials like Microban® to inhibit the growth of microbes in hospitals. We can expect to see an expansion of the use of antimicrobial products in clinics, physicians' offices and long-term care facilities. It is possible to produce antimicrobial concrete by incorporating antimicrobial fibers into concrete, so we may even see medical facilities built entirely of antimicrobial materials.

As is the case with all antimicrobial products, some controversy surrounds the use of antimicrobial plastics. There is concern that triclosan, the chemical most commonly used in antimicrobial toys and cutting boards, can cause health problems in people and lead to the development of antibacterial resistant germs. Both concerns seem to be misplaced. Ciba-Geigy, the company that produces triclosan, has completed studies showing that the compound is non-toxic even when ingested at many times the concentration used in Microban® products. So, even if you eat the whole cutting board, you won't get sick from the triclosan (you may not survive eating all that plastic, though). The US Food and Drug Administration (FDA) also seems to be convinced of the chemical's safety when ingested. It recently approved triclosan for use in toothpaste.

As for antibacterial resistance: in the more than 35 years that antibacterial products containing triclosan have been used by consumers and health professionals, triclosan has never been shown to promote antibacterial or antibiotic resistance. It continues to be effective against a wide range of bacteria, including MRSA.

I'd much rather live in a world with triclosan and other antimicrobials, than one without these useful products.

An exciting new technology makes use of silver to provide effective antimicrobial action that lasts for the lifetime of the plastic. A silver compound is blended into the plastic to suppress the growth of bacteria, algae, fungi, mold, and mildew over the life of the material.

Antimicrobial Synthetic Rubber

A new type of synthetic rubber kills bacteria and other pathogens on contact. The rubber has proved effective in laboratory tests against *Staphylococcus aureus* and other germs that cause hospital infections. The technology incorporates a chemical structure called N-halamine into the polystyrene molecules found in a variety of synthetic rubber materials. N-halamines contain a receptor that binds chlorine atoms. Germs are killed when they come into contact with the surface of the rubber, where they are exposed to the chlorine. It is effective against viruses, fungi and bacteria. The rubber's ability to kill germs can be renewed by soaking it in bleach, which replaces the chlorine atoms. The material can be used in hospitals for patients who are at increased risk for deadly infections due to weakened immune systems. Condoms made of antimicrobial rubber can help prevent the spread of sexually transmitted diseases. Other applications include medical supplies; for example, surgical gloves, aprons and catheters, and consumer products like beverage and food containers, lids and seals, nipples for babies' bottles and pacifiers.

Antimicrobial Clothes

The past five years saw a dramatic growth in the availability of antimicrobial clothing. Manufacturers have developed a new generation of high-performance fabrics that incorporates technology to effectively inhibit the growth of bacteria and other micro-organisms.

Bacteria can cause unpleasant odours in clothes and footwear, and can lead to skin infections. Fungal growth in clothes and socks can cause infections like athlete's foot and jock itch. By inhibiting microbial growth in clothing, we can reduce the likelihood of odours and skin infections.

Initially, antimicrobial fabrics were used mainly for sport and outdoor wear, but the technology is rapidly being incorporated in all lines of clothing, from travel and work wear to casual clothing.

Several new technologies are used to manufacture antimicrobial fabrics, including silver, antibacterial chemicals like triclosan and N-halamines.

Silver is one of the oldest known antimicrobial agents and is effective against more than 650 strains of destructive and odour-causing bacteria, yeast, fungi and mold. Treating fabrics with silver is one of the safest and most effective ways to create antimicrobial clothing. Silver is bonded permanently to fabrics in a coating process or embedded during synthetic fiber manufacture. The use of silver-treated clothing is growing in the food industry, in health institutions and other sterile workplaces.

Fabrics treated with *antimicrobial chemicals* such as triclosan can provide protection against odour-causing bacteria, mold and mildew. Before the introduction of Microban®, chemical treatments remained effective for a relatively short time because the chemicals washed out. Microban® engineered a manufacturing process that binds triclosan directly to plastic fibers. The result is continuous antimicrobial protection for the useful life of the fabric. Microban® has become the chemical treatment of choice for socks, footwear, active wear, sports equipment and linen.

N-halamines are chemical structures that contain disease-fighting chlorine. When bacteria, viruses and other germs come into contact with the N-halamine compound, they are killed within minutes. Welding the N-halamine compound to fabric is not much different from the process the textile industry uses to create wrinkle-free garments. The treatment will last through about five launderings and can be re-activated by adding chlorine bleach to the rinse cycle or soaking the garment in a chlorine bleach solution.

The technology can be used effectively for a wide range of applications including active wear, socks, diapers, sheets, dishcloths, protective clothing for healthcare workers, hospital sheets, and patient gowns. N-halamine treated fabrics are also being tested by military scientists for effectiveness in protecting against biological and chemical weapons.

An interesting *new technology* developed by research scientists deploys tiny molecular 'daggers' that may be used to make microbe-killing clothes. The daggers, which are attached to fabric fibers in a solution, cut the fatty membranes of bacteria and fungal spores; the charged ends of the daggers then disrupt delicate bonds within the pathogens. In early tests, culinary yeast and candida have been destroyed. Eventually, the technology could be tailored to create antifungal socks, and even military uniforms that can destroy anthrax and other biological agents on contact.

Magic (Silver) Bullet?

'Every germ cloud has a silver lining.'

Silver provides antimicrobial protection that prevents the growth of bacteria and fungi. The use of silver to control the growth of micro-organisms dates back to the time of the Roman Empire, and silver has been used for centuries in everything from jewellery and eating utensils to wound-care products. Silver containers have been used to keep their contents from spoiling for centuries. Early American settlers put silver dollars in milk to prevent spoilage. Research into the ability of silver to inhibit the growth of bacteria began in the late 19th century. Today there is growing recognition that silver-based antimicrobial technology can be used safely and effectively.

A number of silver-based pharmaceutical products, including wound dressings and treatments for eye infections were introduced over the past several decades, many of which are still in use. However, the cost of silver and the technical challenges of processing the metal into the ultra-fine particles necessary for optimum performance limited its use in over-the-counter treatments and other consumer products.

Recent innovations in silver technology have led to the introduction of more and affordable silver-based products to prevent and treat infections, including silver-impregnated plastic bandages; silver solutions that can be sprayed on burns, open wounds or other surfaces; silver-impregnated antimicrobial plastic; silver-treated antimicrobial steel; and silver-infused bandages for the treatment of serious burn wounds.

Recently developed compounds contain silver ions that interact with humidity in the air to continually suppress the growth of bacteria, mold, mildew, fungi and other microbes.

Silver-based compounds can be used in appliances, building products, food processing and packaging, heating and air conditioning equipment, medical devices, water filtration and delivery systems, pens, brushes, bank cards, promotional items, textiles, touch screens, and many other applications. The compounds have been used successfully in plastic films and moulded parts, fibers and fabrics, and coatings for metals. It can also be applied to installed equipment and existing facilities.

Steel and appliance makers are joining the battle against bacteria with antimicrobial doorknobs and appliances. There is even a germ-free house near Los Angeles to show what the future may hold. The house in Simi Valley features stainless steel surfaces and appliances coated with a silver-based antimicrobial compound, that, in addition to killing germs, also makes cleaning easier than traditional stainless steel.

Ultraviolet Light

Ultraviolet rays will kill most germs, including *Salmonella, E. coli, Streptococcus, Staphylococcus*, hepatitis, and many other bacteria and viruses that cause infectious diseases. The US Centers for Disease Control and Prevention (CDC) has recommended ultraviolet disinfection to eliminate disease-causing germs for more than 40 years.

Ultraviolet light is being used in a growing number of applications, ranging from commercial water purifiers to pocket-sized instruments that use ultraviolet radiation to kill a wide range of germs. Ultraviolet light can safely sanitize toothbrushes, telephones, remote controls, toilet seats and flushing handles, computer mice, keyboards and mouse pads, children's toys, doorknobs, ABM touch screens and many other surfaces. Ultraviolet lighting installed in heating, ventilation, and air conditioning systems can dramatically reduce building-related illness. Tests have shown that ultraviolet germicidal irradiation (UVGI) can reduce the concentrations of microbial organisms and endotoxins in ventilation systems by as much as 99%.

Food Irradiation

Food irradiation kills bacteria in food with radiation. Irradiation works like an X-ray, but instead of taking a picture, the food is exposed to a radioactive beam. Any bacteria and other germs on the food are killed within seconds, and the food is sterilized. The process can prevent public health crises like mass *E. coli* outbreaks caused by contaminated raw meat and poultry products.

Although the technology is increasingly used in many countries, it is controversial. Nobody denies that the process effectively kills germs, but some scientists are concerned that irradiation can damage the genetic make-up of food and cause health problems in humans. However, many researchers and regulatory bodies endorse its safety, stating that there is no evidence that it is unsafe. Some food producers in the US have been using irradiation for more than a decade. In my opinion food irradiation is here to stay. A few years from now, most people will consume irradiated beef and poultry without giving it a second thought.

NEW TECHNOLOGY TO THE RESCUE?

Market forces dictate that the number and variety of products and services that provide protection against germ infection will continue to grow. Many businesses will also have to change the way they operate, in order to protect their customers from harmful germs. Airlines will have to improve hygiene and bio-safety on their aircraft to remain competitive; cruise ship operators will have to put better safeguards in place to prevent outbreaks of infectious illnesses aboard cruise ships; and grocery stores and food service outlets will have to clean up their act to stay competitive. Customers will increasingly take cleanliness and health concerns into account when they decide where to spend their money.

Companies that manufacture hygiene and cleaning products can play an important role to educate consumers on preventing infectious disease. Governments have a responsibility to promote common sense preventive hygiene practices and to implement and enforce appropriate public health regulations.

One thing won't change: You are responsible for protecting yourself against infectious disease.

Stay healthy, stay clean.

Index

Abdominal infections 119
AIDS 7, 15, 84, 153, 206, 225, 230, 262
Air cleaner 82, 211
Air dry 40, 59, 62, 65, 124, 150, 165, 174, 178, 255
Air dryer 29, 30, 46, 74
Airborne germs 50, 86, 112, 116, 142, 204, 210
Aircraft 129, 130, 137, 139, 142, 196
Aircraft toilets 140
Airlines 277
Airport 21, 93, 129, 135, 136, 139, 144
Alcohol 30, 38, 46, 48, 82, 113, 115, 132, 143, 170, 178, 189, 211, 243, 244, 255
Alcohol wipes 36, 79, 170, 172, 174
American Society for Microbiology 21
Amoebic dysentery 44
Animal bites, scratches 229, 233
Animal dander 211
Animal waste 25, 126, 128, 183, 210, 222
Animals 70, 139, 153, 154, 163, 174, 177, 183, 209, 217, 222-227, 234, 262
Anthrax 273

Antibacterial soap 31-32, 89, 115, 164, 213, 221, 233
Antibacterial wipes 30, 39, 48, 111, 123, 134, 170, 178
Antibiotic 7, 115, 121, 154
Antibiotic-resistant bacteria 8
Antifungal 124, 168, 172, 273
Antimicrobial clothing 271
Antimicrobial plastic 267, 268
Antimicrobial rubber 270
Athlete's foot 122, 172, 271
Athletic wear 267
Automated Banking Machines 92, 95, 136
Backcountry 157, 158, 173, 195
Backpacking 54, 174
Bacteria 15, 38-39, 43, 48, 55, 57-59, 79, 82, 90-93, 97, 100, 104, 114, 125, 129, 147, 150, 157, 170, 174, 185, 189, 196, 202, 208, 210, 236, 252, 257, 262
Baking soda 124, 207
Band-aid 38
Bartonella henselae 230
Bathroom 12, 27, 40, 43, 46, 116, 119, 127, 145, 202, 203, 205, 211, 213, 221
Benzalkonium chloride 30
Benzethonium chloride 30
Biodegradable soap 169, 173

INDEX

Bio-safety 277
Bird flu 10
Birds 163, 225
Black Death 244
Bleach 40, 57, 62, 65, 163-165, 173, 188, 191, 202, 205, 215, 217, 260, 271
Blisters 119, 171
Blood 25, 85, 100
Blood transfusion 154
Bloodborne disease 206
Bloodstream infections 115, 119
Boarding pass 136, 137
Body fluids 25, 52, 85, 176, 205, 206
Boil 114, 119
Bottled water 148, 185
Botulism 252, 253
Brain abscess 230
Broken glass 68, 161, 262
Bronchiolitis 44
Bronchitis 104
Bubonic plague 8, 9
Buffet 61, 132, 156
Burns 14, 37, 39, 73, 74, 112, 142, 153, 274
Bus 83, 84, 129, 132
Cafeteria 54, 55, 66
Calicivirus 69
Camping 80, 157, 168, 190
Camping shower 170
Campylobacter 69, 101, 208, 252

Candida 273
Car 30, 56, 81
Carbolic acid 49, 113
Carpet deodorizer 207
Cat litter 222, 238
Catheter 121
Cat-holes 179
Cats 218, 244
Cat-scratch disease 230
Chain of infection 52, 105, 144, 264, 266
Checkout 39, 99, 103, 106, 216, 266
Chemical disinfection 189
Chicken 70, 107, 136, 140, 147, 202
Chicken pox 44
Chlamydia psittaci. 225
Chlorine 59, 126, 189
Cholera 7, 14, 43, 146, 149, 150, 236, 259
Citrobacter 115
Cleaning cloth 14, 25, 201, 203, 204
Cleaning products 58
Clinic 108, 131, 269
Clostridium difficile 114
Clothes 214
Cockroaches 208, 236, 257
Coffee 46, 91, 139, 147, 151
Coffee maker 91
Cold 12, 21, 23, 31, 44, 73, 79, 85, 90, 92, 132, 265
Coliform 43, 101, 139, 199

INDEX

Colorado tick fever 237, 241
Compost 239, 257
Computer 89, 92, 97, 98, 119
Condom 161, 271
Contact lenses 25, 187
Contaminated food 14, 67, 69, 73, 78, 132, 146, 216, 254
Contaminated water 70, 125, 179
Cooler box 56, 78, 163, 165
Coughing 25, 35, 74, 93, 112, 127, 135, 156, 172, 175, 210, 264
Countertop 40, 69, 72, 75, 145, 161, 165, 206, 269
Cream 71, 77, 147
Credit cards 137, 265
Cross-contamination 60, 75
Crowds 35, 155
Cruise ship 23, 131, 155, 277
Cryptosporidiosis 146, 147
Cryptosporidium 69, 125, 186, 189, 192, 252
Cupboard 203, 207
Cutlery 61, 62, 64, 77, 79, 149
Cuts 11, 14, 37, 73, 112, 142, 153, 157, 170, 206, 253
Cutting board 14, 58, 60, 62, 256, 268, 270
Dairy 56, 104, 107, 118, 136, 140, 147, 216, 258
Day care centres 32
DDT 7
DEET 240, 242, 246, 247

DEET Alternatives 249
Defrost 60
Dehydration 169
Deli 54, 55, 107
Dengue fever 239
Dental hygiene 162, 172
Deposit envelope 96
Desk 91
Detergent 61, 64, 91, 124, 184, 188, 201, 209, 215, 223
Dettol 178
Developing countries 68, 129, 147, 150, 154, 182, 185
Deworming 223
Diaper 25, 106, 127, 205, 215
Diarrhea 8, 10, 21, 69, 71, 90, 114, 125, 127, 150, 169, 175, 183, 203, 226
Dining car 132
Dishcloth 40, 63, 69, 273
Dishes 26, 40, 60, 64, 68, 73, 77, 145, 163, 165, 170, 173, 201, 219, 227
Dishwasher 40, 61, 63, 65, 89
Disinfectant 30, 34, 38, 57, 102, 113, 119, 126, 143, 154, 170, 177, 201, 205, 217, 223, 228, 243, 244
Disinfectant spray 49, 89, 94, 134, 145
Disinfectant wipes 81, 85, 89, 134, 138, 145, 221
Distilled water 195
Doctors' offices 35, 108, 131

INDEX

Dog waste 161, 222, 258, 262
Dogs 217, 222, 238, 244
Doorhandle 14, 23, 29, 40, 46, 51, 94, 145, 156, 166, 176, 201, 207
Doorknob 23, 37, 46, 53, 95, 111, 204, 275
Drain 25, 52, 63, 213, 268, 269
Drinking fountain 136
Drinking water 39, 90, 130, 139, 148, 175, 182, 197
Drug-resistant bacteria 32, 119, 269
Dust 14, 82, 163, 205, 211, 231, 253, 255
Dysentery 10, 14, 43, 70, 92, 95, 146, 236, 238, 257, 259
E. coli 8, 39, 43, 69, 70, 95, 100, 103, 106, 115, 122, 125, 146, 154, 167, 182, 208, 234, 252, 257, 259, 262, 275
E. hirae 39
Ear infection 114, 125
Ebola virus 7
Eggs 56-58, 60, 65, 69, 77, 107, 130, 136, 202
Elevator 23, 100, 137
Encephalitis 239, 244
Entamoeba histolytica 44
Enterobacter 115
Enterobius vermicularis 44
Enterococcus faecalis 100, 269
ESBL-producing bacteria 115

Escalator 23, 137
Ethyl alcohol 30, 49, 82, 113, 211
Exotic pets 218
Expiry date 56
Eye drops 138, 142
Eye infection 125, 274
Face mask 86, 112, 134, 142, 255, 265
Farm animals 154, 183, 234
Faucet 29, 46, 89, 100, 119, 120, 139, 141, 145, 166, 188, 206, 213, 221
FDA 270
Fecal contamination 43
Fecal matter 100, 146, 150
Fecal strep 101
Feces 43, 71, 80, 92, 126, 176, 179, 206, 209, 224, 236
Feet 123, 124, 167, 170, 171
Filariasis 239
First aid kit 134, 153, 181, 190
Fish 26, 56, 60, 71, 75, 146, 202, 253
Fleas 224, 243
Flesh-eating disease 8, 95, 115
Flies 164, 166, 174, 178, 205, 208, 236, 257, 262
Floor 26, 43, 51, 53, 72, 75, 85, 122, 138, 200, 205, 221
Flu 14, 21, 31, 35, 40, 44, 48, 52, 73, 79, 85, 90, 103, 108, 112, 118, 122, 132, 265

INDEX

Fomites 93
Food irradiation 276
Food poisoning 202, 208, 237
Food safety 54, 66, 72, 78, 89, 106, 117, 130, 133, 139, 146, 158, 162, 216
Food service 40, 54, 67, 72, 77, 116, 266, 277
Food waste 174, 262
Foodborne illness 54, 60, 67, 72, 78, 130, 163
Footwear 214, 271
Freezer 57, 167
Fridge 57, 167, 203, 207, 216
Frozen food 57, 60
Fruit 59, 69, 118, 134, 147, 149, 151, 202, 256
Fungal infection 122, 124, 167
Fungi 11, 15, 32, 38, 49, 82, 93, 113, 122, 129, 157, 172, 178, 207, 211, 217, 218, 252, 257, 268, 271, 273
Game consoles 207
Garbage 10, 26, 73, 75, 89, 160, 163, 170, 177, 183, 202, 208, 220, 227, 233, 238, 261, 263
Gardening 25, 213, 243, 252, 254, 255
Gastroenteritis 209, 257, 259
Gastrointestinal illness 71, 155
Germ Etiquette 264
Germ-free house 275

Germicidal rinse 171
Giardia 44, 69, 125, 175, 179, 184, 189, 193, 195, 252
Giardiasis 44, 146, 147, 150
Gloves, disposable 61, 74, 86, 116, 134, 137, 188, 194, 206, 228, 263
Grilling 60
Groceries 56
Grocery store 56, 99-101, 103, 148, 265, 277
Guesthouse 145
Guests 220
Gym 122
Haemolytic Uremic Syndrome 71, 100, 234
Hand sanitizer 30, 39, 85, 89, 96, 98, 102, 105, 116, 123, 134, 137, 144, 156, 162, 171, 178, 221, 234, 265
Hantavirus 227
Hazardous foods 62, 65
Health authority 73, 78
Health Canada 186, 187
Healthcare 116, 117, 120, 266, 273
Heart infection 100, 230
Heating 201
HEPA filter 112, 211
Hepatitis 10, 48, 84, 131, 149, 153, 262, 275
Hepatitis A 14, 21, 30, 44, 69, 71, 90, 100, 146, 155
Hepatitis B 15, 206

INDEX

Hepatitis E 44
Herpes 15, 106
Hiking 168, 172, 176, 248
HIV/AIDS 15, 153, 206, 225, 230, 262
Home distiller 195
Hospital 32, 39, 97, 113-118, 120, 131, 154, 268, 271
Hospital food 116
Hospital washrooms 118
Hospital-acquired infection 113, 121, 123, 269
Hot tub 127, 128
Hotel 43, 131, 144, 148
Human waste 179
Hydrogen peroxide 38, 49, 113, 255, 256
Hypodermic needles, syringes 84, 134, 154
Ice 148
Indalone 246
In-hospital infections 115
Insect repellent 134, 164, 178, 181, 240, 244, 246, 247
Insect screen 164, 181
Insect-borne disease 7, 8, 236, 245
Insecticide 238, 240, 244
Insects 9, 58, 162, 166, 174, 177, 179, 180, 212, 219, 236, 237, 245, 250, 257
Iodine 38, 189, 190, 194, 244
Irradiated beef, poultry 276
Jaundice 44, 71

Jock itch 271
Kidney disease 71, 100, 234
Kitchen 40, 58, 63, 89, 161, 164, 202, 267
Klebsiella pneumoniae 115
Lakes 125, 128
Laundry 214
Leftover food 61, 163, 174, 220
Legionnaire's disease 8, 155
Lemon eucalyptus, oil of 250
Libraries 97
Listeria 257, 208
Litter 84, 161, 261
Litter box 25
Luggage cart 137
Lunch room 89
Lung abscess 230
Lyme disease 8, 227, 236, 237, 241
Mad cow disease 8
Magazines 111, 137, 139
Mail 25
Make-up 25, 36, 106
Malaria 7, 9, 10, 15, 236, 237, 239
Marburg fever 8
Mattress covers 268
Measles 14, 44, 155
Meat 14, 26, 56, 58, 61, 69, 70, 75, 77, 100, 106, 107, 118, 130, 136, 146, 151, 156, 167, 202, 215, 258, 276
Medical emergency 131, 154

INDEX

Medical facilities 108, 131, 154, 269
Medical products 267
Meeting room 89
Meningitis 8, 10, 21, 90, 114, 155, 230
Methicillin 114
Methicillin-resistant Staphylococcus aureus 15, 114, 119, 123, 269
Mice 224, 228, 244, 257, 262
Microban 267, 268
Microfilters 186, 192, 194
Microwave 40, 60, 63, 203
Mildew 268, 270, 272, 274
Milk 69, 70, 147, 151, 274
Mold 66, 124, 164, 205, 207, 211, 268, 270, 272, 274
Money 25, 46, 96, 105, 137
Morganella 115
Mosquito net 181, 240, 248
Mosquitoes 164, 178, 240, 247, 249, 259
Motor vehicles 81
MRSA 15, 114, 119, 123, 269
Mucous membranes 14, 47, 156
Mucus 100
Mumps 44
Municipal water 185, 192, 195
N,N-diethyl-m-toluamide 247
Nails 27, 74, 115, 171, 222
Nasal spray 138, 142

Necrotizing fasciitis 115
Needle 84, 85, 114, 134, 161
New technology 267, 270, 273
N-halamine 270, 272
Norwalk virus 21, 69, 90, 132
NSF International 194
Ocean 125, 128, 169
Odour 82, 170, 207, 271
Outbreak 7, 8, 10, 23, 60, 67, 78, 86, 115, 122, 125, 132, 155, 178, 182, 235, 276
Outdoor wear 267, 271
Packaged food 57, 78, 107
Paper towels 30, 46, 52, 58, 89, 203, 221
Papilloma virus 37, 123
Parakeets 225
Parasites 8, 11, 32, 38, 42, 68, 125, 130, 157, 175, 182, 189, 191, 193, 217, 218, 222, 224, 237, 252, 258
Parks 224, 261
Parrots 225
Passports 136
Pasteurellosis 229
Penicillin 115
Permethrin 242, 246
Pest control 208, 220, 244
Pets 25, 203, 217, 222, 242
Pharmacies 38, 104, 190
Phenol 49, 82, 113, 211
Picaridin 250
Picnic 61, 149
Pink eye 104, 106

INDEX

Pinworm 44
Pit toilets 176
Plague 8, 9, 227, 244
Plantar warts 123
Plastic bandage 38, 138, 143, 153, 274
Play areas 111
Pneumonia 8, 10, 44, 100, 114, 119, 127, 230
Polio 14
Pool 126, 160
Poultry 26, 56, 58, 60, 75, 77, 100, 107, 202, 215, 276
Preventive hygiene 12, 15, 143, 266, 277
Preventive medication 11
Protective clothing 180, 273
Proteus 115
Protozoa 150, 192
Pseudomonas aeruginosa 39, 115, 119, 127
Pseudomonas sp 229
Psittacosis 225
Public telephones 93, 136
Public toilet 23, 44, 48, 100
Public transportation 25, 83, 85, 132, 144
Public washroom 22, 26, 28, 33, 39, 42, 44, 46, 51, 89, 119, 132, 156, 167, 177
Purse 49, 51, 112
Pyrethroid coils 240
Quaternary ammonium 48, 49, 113

Rabies 153, 227, 232
Raccoons 227, 229
Rats 208, 228, 244, 257, 262
Reading glasses 85
Recontamination 29, 51, 89
Recreational facilities 122
Recreational water illness 125
Refrigerator 56, 57, 60, 89, 163, 167, 216
Reptiles 218, 223, 226
Respiratory illness 21, 93, 125, 155
Restaurant 32, 44, 54, 66, 97
Restroom 21, 95
Reverse osmosis 186, 192, 194, 196
Rift Valley fever 239
Ringworm 209
River 125, 126, 128, 169, 172, 185, 192, 245, 262
Rocky Mountain Spotted Fever 227
Rodents 9, 58, 162, 163, 212, 219, 227, 229, 244
Rotavirus 44, 100, 146
Rubella 44, 155
Rutgers 612 246
RWIs 125, 127
Salad 60, 70, 147, 151, 167
Saliva 25, 35, 79, 84, 92, 100, 229, 230, 237
Salmonella 8, 43, 69, 101, 115, 225, 226, 252
Salmonellosis 14, 69, 146, 225

INDEX

Sandbox 209, 224
Sanitizing wipes 102, 106, 171
SARS 8, 21, 23, 115
Savlon 178
Scarlet fever 44
School 32, 44, 48
School bus 84
Schoolbag 51
Seafood 56, 58, 65, 77, 100, 107, 118, 130, 136, 147, 149, 156, 203, 215, 258
Septicemia 15, 131
Sexual contact 15, 153
Sexually transmitted diseases 153
Shellfish 146, 151, 156
Shigella 43, 69, 125
Shigellosis 70, 146
Shopping 25, 35, 46, 56, 99, 102, 104, 137, 152, 212
Shopping basket 99
Shopping cart 99, 101, 103
Shopping mall 48, 94
Shower 119, 145, 167, 204,
Silver 39, 270, 272, 273
Sink 43, 51, 62, 74, 89, 145, 165, 196, 204, 227
Skin infection 119, 125, 271
Smallpox 44
Sneezing 25, 93, 172, 210, 264
Soap 22, 26, 31, 34, 46, 58, 74, 141, 164, 170, 202, 213, 255, 265

Soap dispenser 52, 74, 141, 213
Social customs 130
Socks 124, 138, 172, 242, 268, 271-273
Soil 69, 179, 197, 231, 234, 252, 255
Spa 127
Spills 58, 59, 76, 82, 85, 126, 204, 205
Sponge 59, 62
Stagnant water 120, 220, 259
Staph infection 114, 119
Staph. aureus 39, 95, 100, 229
Stethoscope 113
Stomach flu 52
Street market 152
Street vendors 148, 149
Strep 10, 44, 95, 114
Streptococcus 44, 100, 114, 122, 229
Subway 83, 84, 87, 145
Superbug 114
Supermarkets 100, 101, 102
Surgery 109, 112, 121
Surgical gloves 271
Swimming 125
Syringe 134, 154
Tabletop 145, 165, 216
Take-out food 54, 66, 77
Tampon 25
Tap 74, 120, 136, 143, 145, 147, 188, 192, 213
Tap water 120, 145, 184, 192

INDEX

Tapeworm 244
Taxi 83, 145
Tea 139, 147
Telephones 46, 89, 92, 207
Tetanus 12, 15, 231, 252, 255, 257, 262
Tick bite 237, 243
Ticket dispenser 97
Ticks 169, 181, 236, 241
Tinea, tinea pedis 122
Toilet 43, 46, 52, 89, 132, 145, 176, 204, 269
Toilet seat cover 47, 89, 221
Toiletries 216
Toothbrush 36, 138, 172, 180, 204, 268, 275
Towel 28, 62, 123, 138, 145, 165, 180, 204, 215, 265
Toxic shock syndrome 119
Toxin 114, 174, 231, 253, 276
Toxoplasmosis 223, 224
Toys 40, 111, 265, 267, 276
Trachoma 236
Train 87, 129, 132
Travel 9, 11, 31, 39, 129, 182
Traveler's diarrhea 129, 150
Triclocarban 32
Triclosan 31, 32, 267, 269, 272
Tuberculosis 8, 14, 127, 237
Tularemia 241, 244
Typhoid 7, 10, 43, 146, 149, 236, 244, 257, 259
Ultraviolet light 186, 193, 275
Ultraviolet purifiers 196

Upholstery 82, 207, 221
Urinal 43, 52
Urinary tract infection 115, 119
Urine 52, 100, 176, 222
US Centers for Disease Control and Prevention 20, 54, 123, 275
Vaccination 12, 156
Vacuuming 82, 200, 205, 244
Vancomycin 115
Vancomycin-resistant Enterococci 115, 119
Varicella 155
Vector 157, 236, 241
Vegetables 59, 69, 104, 135, 147, 149, 151, 202, 256
Vending machines 97, 136, 137, 196
Veterinarian 219, 223, 224, 232, 233, 244
Vibrios 43
Virus 15, 68, 130, 194, 211
Vomit 25, 69, 71, 112, 206, 241
VRE 115, 119
Waiting room 35, 39, 108, 109, 111
Walkerton 182
Washroom 21, 22, 48, 50, 75, 106, 111, 117, 118, 124, 127, 137, 159, 161, 167
Wastebin 203, 208
Water bottles 124, 135, 180, 197

INDEX

Water contamination 180
Water cooler 91, 187, 188
Water features 259
Water filters 39, 192, 194
Water pollution, sources 182
Water purifiers 39, 193, 195
Water, boiling 189, 148, 189, 191, 194, 195
Water, chemical treatment 189, 191
Water, storing 197
Waterborne diseases 147, 182
Waterpark 126

Well 182, 185, 192, 196, 199
West Nile virus, disease 8, 236, 239
Wild animals 227
Wilderness camping 168
Workout equipment 122
Workplace 44, 88, 90
Wound 14, 25, 39, 127, 143, 157, 229, 231, 233, 253, 267, 274
Wound dressing 38, 274
Wound infection 125, 267
Yellow fever 7, 9, 239